COMMUNITY HEALTH CARE

Claire Johnston
and
Kate Brown

First edition 1991
Reprinted 1992
Second edition 1993
Reprinted 1994, 1995

Published by
Macmillan Magazines Ltd
Porters South
4-6 Crinan Street
London N1 9XW

Companies and representatives throughout the world

Printed in Great Britain by
Barwell Colour Print Ltd
Bath, England

ISBN 0-333-626-354

Contents

Throughout this module the personal pronoun 'she' will be used where the subject's gender is not specified. This is for convenience and is not intended to imply gender bias, which we have taken care to avoid.

Introduction

The purpose of this module

This module is one of the three specialist modules –

• *Care of the Mother and Newborn*
• *Mental Health and Mental Handicap*
• *Community Health Care*

— which form part of the *Nursing Times* Open Learning Conversion Programme.

In line with European Community Directives, and in order to register as a first-level nurse on Part 1 of the UKCC register, your pre-registration education and training must include a minimum in theory and practice of:

• 60 hours — Community care
• 150 hours — Care of the mother and newborn
• 150 hours — Mental health and mental handicap.

Each one of the three modules can be used on its own for professional updating, or integrated into other programmes as and when appropriate.

The *Community Health Care* module and your related experience are not intended to turn you into an expert on nursing in the community. However, the experience you gain will enable you to develop an understanding of the health needs of the community and the effects of the care provided in the community on clients and on their carers, and will increase your knowledge of the providers of care in the community, be they from public or voluntary sector services or the client's immediate family or friends.

How to use this module

How and when you gain your experience of community health care will depend on your tutor/counsellor and the relevant nursing managers. However, we do recommend that you work through the first two Sections of *Community Health Care* before you start *Care of the Mother and Newborn* and *Mental Health and Mental Handicap,* as these Sections contain useful information on demography and its relationship with the provision of care.

Throughout this module you will be asked to seek the opinions of various people to help you work through some of the Activities. It may save time and disappointment if you identify at least some of these people, from a variety of age groups, at the beginning of the module and ask their permission to consult them from time to time.

Because you may gain your practical experience in a variety of creative ways, such as following some clients into the community where they will continue to receive care, it is likely that your experience will be spread over quite a long period. You will therefore have the opportunity to talk to a wide range of people, including clients and their carers, during this time.

This practical experience will enable you to see the way in which the resources available for the provision of support and care for clients in the community are organised.

The material in the three specialist modules contains more work than the UKCC minimums specified above for first-level registration. However, you may find that by dovetailing some aspects of the project work, based on the community profile (see below) you can be working on more than one module at the same time. The student notes that accompany these modules give more guidance on planning and managing this work.

The Community Profile

Throughout the three modules, *Community Health Care*, *Care of the Mother and Newborn* and *Mental Health and Mental Handicap*, you will be asked to include in your community profile relevant information you obtain from some of the Activities you undertake.

Do not confuse the community profile with your personal professional profile from the Profile Pack. It is an entirely separate document.

The community profile will provide a record — a picture — of the community in which you and your clients/patients live and work, in particular:

• The people who make up the community
• Their health, social and cultural needs
• The resources and services available to meet those needs.

If you live and work in a large urban area, your community profile may represent only a part of a larger community. However, if you live and work in a rural area, you may be able to develop a picture of a much larger section of the community, if not the entire community.

Whatever your practice setting or specialism, the community profile should become a very useful resource for you.

As the profile grows, it will enable you to demonstrate your developing knowledge and understanding of the community and your client/patient group. It will also offer a point of reference to illustrate any changes which occur, especially in resources and services, as well as your increasing ability to understand the possible effects of these changes on you and your clients/patients.

Building your community profile

Where do you keep it?
You may wish to keep your community profile in a section of your

Student Pack binder. Alternatively, you may find it more convenient to keep it in a separate binder altogether.

How do you keep it?
You are free to develop the profile as you wish, creating sections or categories that best meet your learning objectives.

However, one suggestion is that you divide it into the sections we described above, namely:

• *The people* — looking at the different cultural, religious and social groups; where and at what many of them work; how supportive they are of each other; and, in particular, those who make up your client/patient group.

• *The health and social needs of the community* — again looking at your particular group, or the community as a whole.

• *The resources and services available to meet those needs* — for example, shopping, transport, leisure and sporting facilities, and health, voluntary and social services.

You may decide to expand on these sections, subdivide them, or create entirely different ones.

However you create it, the profile should give you the information you need to help you.

SYMBOLS

The following information will explain the symbols that accompany the Activities in this module. The times given for each of the Activities are approximate only and are intended to reflect the actual time spent with an individual, or reading information. They also include the time spent making notes. The time it takes to locate the people or information you need will undoubtedly vary enormously and would therefore be impossible to estimate.

Some of the Activities in the module ask you to do practical things, which you may not be able to complete during the period you are working on a particular Section. To help you organise your time you should make a rough timetable of when you aim to do them and whether you need to make any arrangements in advance.

Your diary is your own private record of your course work. Use it to make notes of your own ideas and opinions about the work you are doing. You will find it particularly helpful to jot down answers to those Activities with the diary symbol, as these may be used as the basis for discussion or assignment work.

Activities accompanied by this sign are reflective Activities, which ask you to think about a particular point in the text before reading on. You may decide that it would be useful to record these in your diary as well.

A number of the Activities (particularly the Focus Activities at the end of each Section, see below) encourage you to include the material you gather in your community profile. This is designed to help you record your developing knowledge of the community and is therefore a key tool in the work you do for this part of the programme. (See the notes on pages 6 and 7 about building a community profile.)

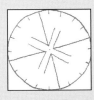

At the end of each Section of the module there is a Focus Activity, which is intended to draw together the ideas and situations you have been exploring, and to relate them to your own experience and locality. There almost certainly will be some written work in the Focus Activity and it may also involve research, review or discussion.

1.Care in the community

In this first Section of the module, we want to explore two issues which are fundamental to any discussion of the community nurse's role:

• How does community nursing differ from hospital nursing?
• What is the nature of the community health-care environment?

The continuum of care

Many nurses still see a sharp division between hospital and community care — two very different types of service. However, in practice, these sharp distinctions are breaking down. Many patients who, a few years ago, would have spent several days as in-patients are now treated in day surgery units and complete their recovery at home. Eight thousand people who would otherwise spend long periods of time in a hospital acute ward receiving treatment (such as intravenous therapy or chemotherapy) are now cared for by home care schemes, or what are known as 'hospital at home' schemes[1].

In some areas, people who fracture their hips are discharged within 24 hours and their care continues at home[2]. In care of the elderly units, length of stay was reduced by 50% in the 10 years to 1992[3].

Since the GP contract of 1990, 68% of GP practices[4] now carry out minor surgery on practice premises. Hospitals, for their part, have made efforts to make the hospital environment more homely and less clinical. For example, care of the elderly units encourage patients to bring in some personal belongings or items of furniture, or the nurses in that department might wear their own clothes instead of uniforms. The midwifery department may make labour rooms more home-like, and less clinical. The outpatient department may provide play facilities in the waiting area.

However, despite the changing nature of provision, the experience of being a patient in a hospital, even a day patient, is still very different from being nursed in the community. When admitted to a hospital, people are known as patients. But, once transferred home, they are often referred to by community nurses as 'clients'.

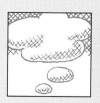

ACTIVITY 1
5 MINS
Why are these two different terms used? What impression do you think they convey about the relotionship between the nurse and the person being cared for?

Patients in hospital are viewed as dependent, passive and usually sick, but the moment they are discharged to the community nursing service they become 'clients' and the power relationship shifts in their favour. Some community nurses consider the word 'clients' an inappropriate term, more appropriate for use by hairdressers or solicitors whose clients choose to employ professionals and to pay for their services. The term used is therefore a statement about the status of the people concerned, although GPs still refer to people who require their services as their 'patients'.

You will find some nurses referring to *consumers*. This is a term which implies active participation, with people exercising choice in health care, including what they get from the community nursing service. Talking about *users* of services has recently gained popularity as the concept of advocacy and people having 'rights' has developed.

Whatever labels are used, there are some fundamental differences between nursing in hospital and nursing in the community:

• The identity of the clients
In a hospital ward, a policeman and a drug dealer may lie side by side but will look the same at first glance because most people look similar in a pair of pyjamas. Both patients are locked into hospital routine and, even when nurses work hard to take account of the facets of a patient's personality and lifestyle, it is not always possible to override hospital routine. In the community, the nurse is a guest in the patient's home, an environment in which the patient, or his carers, hold 'power'. In this environment, the nurse has to build a relationship with all those involved, not just the patient, on their own terms. In fact, it is important to note here that the community nurse needs to regard all these individuals, not only the person receiving care, as clients.

• The identity of the nurses
Most hospital patients will expect a nurse to wear a uniform. It is one of the traditional ways patients identify who nurses are. In the community, health visitors, community psychiatric nurses and, increasingly, district nurses do not wear uniforms. Nurses working in the community generally consider uniforms an unnecessary barrier between themselves and their clients. Nurses do not want to be seen as 'authority' figures by their clients and wearing a uniform sets them apart from other professional colleagues, such as teachers, social workers or probation officers. Of course this approach is not unique to community nurses. In many elderly care environments nurses have discarded their uniforms and there are also acute areas now where nurses are experimenting with a non-uniform policy[5].

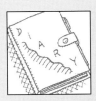

ACTIVITY 2
20 MINS
If you wear a nursing uniform, ask yourself what the benefits are to patients or to you. Write these down. Then include in your diary a brief account of what effects wearing ordinary clothes might have on your nursing practice. How do you think your identity as a nurse might be affected?

Uniforms can have considerable advantages where factors involving easy identification, easy-to-care-for working clothes, cost and professional status are involved, but they have distinct disadvantages when they reinforce unhelpful nurse-client barriers.

If receiving care outside the hospital setting is a different experience, so, indeed, is providing that care.

ACTIVITY 3
30 MINS
Ask three community nurses what they enjoy about nursing in the community and why. Then ask them to compare working in the community to working in hospital. This Activity could be carried out over the period of your community allocation. You need not make a special visit or time to ask these questions – they may take place during a visit for another purpose.

This Activity could generate as many different answers as there are community nurses, but one point community nurses tend to make quite frequently is that they particularly enjoy the opportunity they have to develop a relationship with a client over a period of time. This, in turn, offers greater scope for health promotion than is usual in a hospital setting.

ACTIVITY 4
15 MINS
Consider the following scenario:

Jenni, an energetic two–year–old, has recently been seen in the accident and emergency department having suffered a partial-thickness burn from a gas fire. Both the nurse in the department and the health visitor would be in a position to offer advice and support to prevent a subsequent injury.

• List in your diary any advantages that you think the health visitor might have.

Although the accident and emergency nurse would have the advantage of immediacy and the possible heightened awareness of the parents, this might be outweighed by parental anxiety about Jenni's current injury, and this anxiety might, therefore, interfere with their ability to absorb information. The health visitor would be able to choose a moment after Jenni had returned home, when the immediate shock of the incident had subsided, and her parents would be more receptive to discussion.

Additional advantages that the health visitor might have include:

• A previous established relationship with Jenni's parents
• Awareness of family economic circumstances (purchase of safety equipment, such as fireguards, might be a problem)

- Local knowledge about where to purchase a guard (new or secondhand)
- Opportunity for a home visit/clinic discussion which might indicate other problems. It has been shown that accidents are often indicative of family stress[6].

So we can see that at opposite ends of the health care continuum, hospital and community, there are differences that are fundamental to the nature of the nurse's role, and we will be considering these in further detail as we work through this module.

In the second part of this first Section we want to explore the notion of 'community' itself, and consider the nature of the environment in which community health care takes place.

Understanding the community

Community nursing takes account not only of the client as the individual but also the client in the wider context: the individual's family, and the community in which the client lives.

Knowing the local community and understanding its idiosyncracies is essential for the day-to-day work of the community nurse. For example, she might be looking for complicated reasons as to why nobody came to a Tuesday clinic when the explanation simply may be that people prefer to go to town on market day, which happens to be Wednesday! On a deeper level, knowledge and sensitivity to local custom avoids the pitfall of rushing into action which might offend because of ignorance.

Furthermore, understanding the local community is the starting point for identification of health needs.

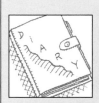

ACTIVITY 5
5 MINS
List a few of the ways you have heard the word 'community' used. In your opinion, does the word 'community' mean the same thing in each instance?

What does the word 'community' mean to you?

There have been many attempts to define the word, but most agree that 'community' implies that the people who form that community have something in common. However, some definitions are more limited and the words 'locality', 'neighbourhood' and 'community' are sometimes used as if they were interchangeable.

Luker and Orr[7] suggest that the concept of community should be examined under the following headings:

1. Community as locality
2. Community as social activity
3. Community as social structure
4. Community as sentiment.

Number 1 is about *place*, numbers 2 and 3 are about *people* and number 4 is about *perception* — how we see our community and how others see it.

An example of 4 would be that some people may have left a particular geographical area years ago but still feel part of that community.

Number 1 is not as straightforward as it appears. Many people feel they live in a community, but have difficulty deciding where it begins and ends geographically and which people it includes.

ACTIVITY 6
10-15 MINS
Think about where you live now. If asked 'Where do you live?', how would you answer?

Jot down what you like and dislike about where you live.

Make this Activity part of your community profile.

Did you find your answers touched on the headings mentioned above or were your answers strictly to do with your personal family life?

When patients are discharged from hospital, especially if they live alone, it is often said that they have a 'support structure' in the local community. In other words, they have connections with local people and organisations who can provide care and support.

Now imagine you were ill. How much support do you think would be available to you where you live?

ACTIVITY 7
5-10 MINS
Find a map of where you live and make a photocopy. Highlight your own home and draw pencil lines to indicate your connections with the community. Include such things as the chemist and the paper shop as well as such 'official' connections as your church or your children's school, for example.

Make this Activity part of your community profile.

You might find that this Activity leaves you feeling a bit disconcerted because you do not seem to have many local connections! This is often the case when people are working full time, because they discover that their life revolves around the workplace. Many first-time mothers who have only recently stopped going out to work also get the same results when they do this Activity at antenatal classes.

Can we assume that because people have connections in the local community these connections are necessarily supportive? It might be useful to repeat Activity 7 for a client that you meet during this module, to see just how extensive the support structure is in that person's case.

Community health profiles

Looking back at Activity 6, did your answers include a mixture of what you felt about where you live and facts about where you live? If it did, then you have the beginnings of what community health workers call a community health profile. Such a profile contains a mixture of *objective* and *subjective* data.

Broadly speaking, objective data include facts and figures about the area, and subjective data involve people's (including the nurses') feelings and opinions about the area.

The data used in a community health profile include those directly related to health and illness (such as mortality figures or immunisation uptake rates) and information about factors that influence health.

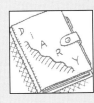

ACTIVITY 8
5 MINS
Using your own experience, write down in your diary a list of the factors that can influence the health of a community.

Among the things you could have noted (with some examples in brackets), might have been:
- Environmental characteristics (pollution)
- The history of the community (such as when drains were installed, lead pipes laid or whether it was a mining or farming community)
- Population characteristics (birth rate)
- Social and economic influences (social class distribution)
- Local organisations (strength of local voluntary organisations)
- Political influence (resources given to health care)
- Significant local people/groups (local campaigns)
- Social services (availability, accessibility)
- Health services (availability, accessibility)
- How the members of the local population perceive their community (they may have a negative view of the housing estate where they live).

Identification of health needs

In compiling their health profiles, community nurses aim to create a practical resource that will help them to identify the specific health needs of their 'patch', the resources available to meet those needs and an awareness of any difficulties which may impede that work.

This aspect of the community nurses' work complements that of health and local authority officers whose specific brief is to assess the health needs of their authority (Fig 1). Under the 1990 NHS and

Community Care Act, all health authorities are required 'to secure measurable improvements in the health of their resident population'. To this end, in England the department of public health of each health authority publishes an annual report on the health of its population and, in addition, publishes detailed documents on the health needs of particular sections of that population. The Family Health Services Authority (FHSA) (or the equivalent in your country), which manages general practitioner services, dentists and pharmacists, commonly contributes to these publications. Furthermore, local authorities, in conjunction with district health authorities (DHAs) or health boards and FHSAs (or the equivalent in your country), are obliged to update their community care plan, which is a public document setting out their strategy.

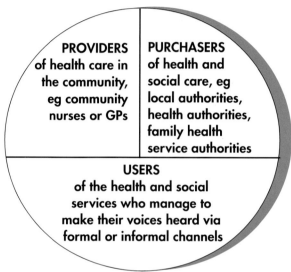

Fig 1. Those involved in identifying health needs in a community

Although the documents and reports published by the various authorities are useful starting points for community nurses, the data are often not detailed enough to produce the sort of profile that will be useful to the nurse in her day-to-day work because a health or local authority might encompass communities with widely differing health needs. So although the nurses often start from the general data of these reports, the wheel comes full circle when they in turn contribute their local knowledge to the DHA to assist future planning.

Making sense of reports and judging which data will be useful for a community health profile takes a little time.

Making sense of data
Reading facts and figures (objective data) about an area that you know well (or thought you knew well!) is often very interesting. Assumptions such as 'I thought nearly everyone had a car', or 'Hardly anyone has an outside toilet these days', can be blown apart suddenly. However, it is very easy to find yourself swimming in statistics. Before you plunge in, there are a few terms with which you should become familiar:
• Demography
• Epidemiology
• Incidence and prevalence.

Demography is the study of whole populations of people, with particular reference to the numbers of people involved (for example: How many people live in a particular area? How old are they? What sex are they? and so on). Most of the basic data come from the census and registrations of births, deaths and marriages.

Many GP practices now have age/sex registers which show the demographic structure of the practice. This allows them to analyse certain factors, such as what percentage of people in their practice are under five years of age, or to identify those patients over 75 years of age who should be screened annually (a condition of the GP contract).

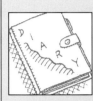

ACTIVITY 9
30-60 MINS
Through your community link person, make an appointment to meet a practice nurse or GP receptionist at a practice that has an age/sex register. Ask them to describe what use the practice makes of the register and then list the benefits of it in your diary.

Epidemiology is not the study of epidemics, although it does include this. It is the study of the distribution and determinants of disease in human populations. In simple terms it tries to answer the questions:

- Who gets ill?
- Why do they get ill?
- How should they be treated?

ACTIVITY 10
15 MINS
Ask your local college librarian for a copy of the annual report on the health of your district. Choose a particular condition (for example, coronary heart disease or HIV/AIDS) and see what information on this topic is included in the annual report of the department of public health of your local health authority or the equivalent in your own country.

Now compare this information about your district with the material that can be found in the document *On the State of the Public Health*, which is published annually by the Department of Health and which should be readily available in college libraries.

How different is your district from the national picture?

Record the differences in your community profile.

When doing Activity 10 you almost certainly came across the words 'incidence' and 'prevalence'.

Incidence is the term used to describe the number of people who begin to suffer from a specific disease in a given time period (for example, how many new cases of AIDS were diagnosed in 1992 in a particular area).

Prevalence is the term used to describe the number of people who actually have a specific disease at a specific time (for example, how many people in a given area had AIDS on June 9, 1992).

The census: an important source of data

Every 10 years the government carries out a full census in the UK. Many of you may remember completing a census form in 1991. The census gives information on key areas, such as:
• The population of an area
• The housing in an area

plus several special topics, many of which are of particular interest to community nurses (for example, types of people moving house, employment and class structure and educational qualifications of the population).

Statistics are available for the nation and for the counties, but the statistics that community nurses often find the most interesting are called the *small area statistics,* which provide information about electoral wards. As these are the most detailed aspects of the census information, they tend to be published last — the data from the 1991 census became available during 1993 and 1994.

ACTIVITY 11
15 MINS
Ask your local librarian for the statistics for the electoral ward in which you live. Choose a set of statistics that might significantly affect health care (for example, the number of households which lack basic amenities — bath, indoor WC, hot and cold water supply).

Make a list of the possible impact on health of this lack of basic amenities. Include this list in your community profile.

Your list probably will have included such problems as food poisoning, difficulties with stoma care, the risk of poorly sterilised baby bottles – in fact, anything in which the need for stringent hygiene in the home plays an important part.

Social class and its effect on health

After Activity 8 we listed a number of factors that can influence health, so why are we now singling out social class? The reason is that we want to look at the research that has been assembled which provides evidence that people's social class has a disproportionate effect on their health compared with other factors. Thus the social class composition of a particular area can give us some indication of the health needs of that area.

Community nurses have long been aware of this. However, since the publication of the report *Inequalities in Health*[8] (known as the Black

Report) in 1980, there has been ample supporting evidence. Then, in 1987, the Health Education Authority[9] published a review of the research in this field since the Black Report, which confirmed the conclusions of Sir Douglas Black. Research by Watt and Ecob[10], contrasting Glasgow and Edinburgh, offered further supporting evidence. To explore the findings of the Black Report and, indeed, many other reports, we need to be aware of the registrar general's classification of social classes.

Since 1875 the population has been divided into broad occupational groups or classes, based on job, income and status. The classifications, together with examples for each, are as follows:

I   Professional (accountant, doctor)
II   Intermediate (manager, school teacher)
IIIn   Skilled non-manual (secretary, clerical worker)
IIIm   Skilled manual (bus driver, builder, coalminer)
IV   Partly skilled (agricultural worker, bus conductor)
V   Unskilled (labourer, cleaner).

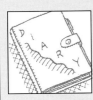

ACTIVITY 12
5 MINS
One of the findings of the Black Report was that children in Social Class V were seven times more likely to die as a result of being knocked down by a car as were children in Social Class I.

List some reasons why you think this is so.

Did your list include availability of safe play areas? For example, do children play in their own garden or do they live on the 14th floor of a tower block? Did you think about how children get to school? Are they driven there or do they make their own way? Did you think about what happens if parents work? Can they afford alternative child care or are children left unsupervised?

The Black Report showed that, despite more than 30 years of the NHS, manual workers and their families still tended to die younger than those in Social Classes I and II, and had much worse health, and, although the health of the nation as a whole has improved (average life expectancy has risen sharply over the past 100 years), the gap between social classes I and V had grown. The report concluded that the main causes of death at a young age (accidents and coronary heart disease) were related to social class.

In practice there were two major implications of the Black Report for nursing in the community. First, could the service as a whole be planned to make the community healthier? Second, could the individual health worker, including the nurse in the community, target her work more effectively to make greater impact on the health needs of individuals or groups of clients?

Looking at social deprivation — its effects on health

In addition to exploring the link between social class and ill health, several attempts have been made to examine whether any particular cluster of factors is associated with increased health need. Rae[11] looked at social deprivation indicators in Glasgow, and Jarman[12] has drawn up a list of factors which can be used to calculate a score for electoral wards as a means of identifying underprivileged areas.

The Jarman Index calculates a score based on the percentage of the following factors in an electoral ward:
• Elderly living alone
• Children under five
• One-parent families
• Unskilled
• Unemployed
• Overcrowded
• Ethnic minorities.

ACTIVITY 13
10-15 MINS

Discuss with one of the community nurses you are in contact with for this module how she identifies the socio-economic factors which have an impact on her clients' health. You might like to ask:

• Does she use any special list or index of factors that help her to identify particular clients as having 'risk' factors?
• Does she look at factual information? (For example, the percentage of the clients in a caseload who are in receipt of income support, or the percentage of children in a school who are eligible for free school dinners)
• Does she base her knowledge on subjective factors? (For example, 'such and such housing estate has a lot of problems')

Enter your findings in your community profile.

How do people feel about the way care is provided in the community?

So far we have concentrated on the objective data that can contribute to a community health profile. Recording objective data can be difficult. If in Activity 10 you chose to look at the amount of information there was on HIV/AIDS in the annual report of the department of public health of your local authority (or the equivalent in your own country) you might already have thought about the limitations of official data. In the case of HIV/AIDS, health planning all over the world has to work with estimated figures for people with the disease.

However, recording *subjective* data, such as how people feel about their community and how they perceive it, can be even more of a problem. This is mainly because the sorts of questions that have to be asked do not always provide answers that can be analysed easily.

For community nurses, such questions might include:
• How many people are socially isolated?
• Is there warmth and closeness?
• Is there a feeling of 'community spirit'?

Making generalisations from individual answers to questions such as these is difficult. But community nurses ignore them at their peril. A good example of this might be: How safe do local residents feel on the street at night?

In fact the actual risk of being the subject of a violent attack in the street in the UK is low — especially compared with our European neighbours. Of course, such a risk does vary from area to area. However, repeated surveys indicate that people (especially women) are reluctant to go out at night[13]. This example is very important if you are a community nurse and plan to hold an evening class or clinic.

Thus, what people think and feel about the area or about the service you offer can be crucial. For this reason many community nurses conduct their own mini-surveys of client views about an aspect of the service as part of their community health profile.

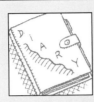

ACTIVITY 14
15 MINS
Note down any recent feedback you have had from clients of yours about aspects of the service you offer. Then consider how you can use this information more systematically as a basis for asking other clients about the issues raised.

There is a link between subjective and objective data; for example, a school nurse may be concerned that the number of children suffering from asthma at a particular school is rising sharply. All those children may be counted somewhere in the statistics or information that may be held about them by their different GPs, but no official figures exist that group those children, and so the data on them, together. The nurse could officially document her local findings and ask for them to be compared with those from other local schools.

Thus, a subjective concern or 'hunch' about something can lead to new questions being asked.

But, don't forget that a community profile is a practical tool. Official figures — especially those collected once a decade — can quickly become out of date. So, community health workers have to rely on their instincts to some extent!

Does the community care? Can it care?

Identifying health needs is one aspect of compiling a community health profile. The other aspect is what *resources* are available to address those health needs.

In the past 15 years the words 'community care' have become part of everyday language and yet we rarely ask, 'What exactly does community care mean?'

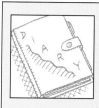

**ACTIVITY 15
10-15 MINS**
Note down in your diary whether you consider that people in the community care about other people as much as they used to.

Although many people might have hospital care for a brief period in their lives, the majority of people never go near a long-stay institution of any kind. Only 5% of people over 65 years of age needing care are in any type of institution[14]. The other 95% are in their own homes — either looking after themselves or being cared for by a relative or friend.

So 95% of the ill and disabled elderly are in the community[14]. But does this mean that the community cares or does it mean that the individual and family struggle to care? Do the individuals being cared for — or the carers — have any choice in the matter? Is care in the community the best option for each individual?

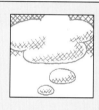

**ACTIVITY 16
10 MINS**
Can you think of any reasons why families may find it hard to care for each other?

You should take into account the following factors:
• The elderly population is increasing while the proportion of people available to provide care is decreasing
• Many of those needing care are aged 85+. Their carers are often 60+. Caring is often a physically demanding job and carers themselves may not be in good health
• Many carers are daughters or sons. However, the increasing trend towards second marriages makes the bonds less clear-cut
• One of the government's responses to unemployment in the 1980s and 1990s has been to encourage young people to work away from home. How does this fit in with also caring for a relative — although, clearly, caring does go on at a distance?
• A government strategy for the 1990s is to encourage women to return to the workforce. Some employers, for example, are increasing the provision of workplace nurseries, but many returners may require a care attendant service for older dependants instead.

Whatever the client group, the demands made on carers by the increasing pressures of age, distance and work will create increasing stress among family, friends and neighbours, despite the official status of, and approval for, community care.

But wait a minute. Don't the words 'community care' mean a bit more than care by families or friends? Do we care for people who are not known personally to us? A cynical view of 'community care' is that it is a 'good thing' unless it is happening in 'my street'. For instance, many planning applications for converting houses or building a new home for people with learning disabilities or people recovering from mental illness have met with local opposition[15]. More recently, units for people suffering with HIV/AIDS have had a similar response.

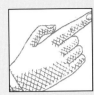

ACTIVITY 17
30-60 MINS
Contact the planning department of your local authority (ask for the Development Control section). Ask if there are any current planning applications for new provision for people with learning disabilities or mental illness in your locality. If so, arrange to visit the department and look at the application and any objections received. Keep an eye on your local paper, too, as these objections are often voiced in letters to the local press.

Another way of looking at whether the wider community cares is to ask what support we give to those who actually do the caring. This will be explored further in Section 4. But there is a more fundamental question, which is often left unasked. Should carers have any choice in whether they care?

The assumption underpinning all recent legislation on community care is that the majority of care will continue to be provided by family, friends and neighbours.

As Jill Pitkeathley, director of the Carers' National Association, has said:

❛ Most carers, it is true, do want to care, but "widening individuals' room for choice" [a reference to the 1990 NHS and Community Care Act] surely means giving them the option to choose not to care ❜ [16]

How far does the state care?
When the term 'community care' was first used, it was frequently said that community care would be cheaper.

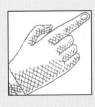

ACTIVITY 18
15-30 MINS
Ask your current manager how much it costs to care for a patient for one day in your clinical area. What is taken into account in arriving at that sum?

At the time community care was initially discussed, figures were widely available for how much it would cost to keep someone in a hospital bed. They seemed large and the assumption was that care in the community would cost less. As a result of this, funding of community care will always be difficult — it involves rationing of scarce resources.

In 1992 a study was published of a disabled client requiring local authority care in the community which demonstrated that a typical client was assessed as needing £120 worth of care a week. However, the local authority care managers had only £41 available for such a client[17].

Defining health needs

In this Section we have already gathered a wealth of information in a community health profile. One of the things which emerges is that identifying health needs is not a straightforward task. Neither is it easy to define a 'need'. A useful way devised by Bradshaw and cited by Ewles and Simnet[18] was to divide it into four categories:

1 *Normative need* This is a need defined by experts or professionals according to their own standards (for example, the need for an immunisation programme for children).
2 *Felt need* This is what people feel they need or want (for example, people may want a night-sitting service to relieve carers).
3 *Expressed need* This is what people say they need (that is, a felt need which has been turned into a request or demand, such as a school crossing following several accidents to children).
4 *Comparative need* This is the difference between two comparable groups (for example, if one health centre has a pharmacy on the premises, people using another health centre without this provision might feel relatively poorly off).

ACTIVITY 19
10 MINS
Using your own experience, identify examples of felt, expressed and comparative health need in your local area. (This could be for where you live or where you work.)

Jot down your thoughts in your community profile.

Once the difficult task of identification of needs is complete, the next hurdle is to contrast these with the resources available. The complicated (and sometimes painful) task of setting priorities of care must be completed first and then health care plans can be formulated.

The other crucial question that has to be faced is at what *level* the identified health care need can be addressed, and by whom? Is an individual, local, national, international or, indeed, global solution required? Can the problem be addressed by the health service or is action on a wider front necessary? (Consider, for example, the alarming rise in skin cancer. At what level can that be addressed?) Community nurses have to decide what their responsibilities are and what they can realistically do. We will look at this further in Section 5.

The Focus Activity for this Section will give you an opportunity to see how the detail of a community profile helps the nurse's awareness of the problems her clients encounter. It is to be hoped that it will also serve as a reminder that hospital and community are not separate worlds; rather, the hospital is one of many community facilities.

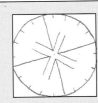

FOCUS
2 HOURS APPROXIMATELY
This Activity asks you to look at the physical access for clients and visitors to your local hospital.

Choose a starting point (such as your own home or the area around a local health centre — preferably somewhere that is for enough away to require transport). First ask in general terms:

- How far do they have to travel?
- What options do they have for getting there?
- What percentage of households in that electoral ward have cars (these data will be in the census report). Remember that not all cars may be available, because of a partner's work commitment, for instance.
- How easy is it to park — and do you have to pay to park? If so, how much?
- How much would a taxi or mini-cab cost?
- How reliable is public transport?
- Who is eligible for hospital transport by ambulance or car?
- What arrangements exist for those with special needs, such as people who use wheelchairs, prams or buggies? (The patients' charters for England, Scotland, Wales and Northern Ireland all state that everyone, including people with special needs, should be able to use services.)

Note your findings in your community profile.

2.Organising care in the community

In Section 1 we looked briefly at the role of the community nurse, and explored the nature of the environment in which she works. As you completed the Activities for that Section, and perhaps began to discuss some of the issues with people who work in community health care, you will have started to build up a profile of your own community (recorded in your community profile) to use as a basis for the rest of this module.

In this second Section we consider how care is organised in the community. We start by looking at the concept of primary health care.

What is primary health care?

We are all familiar with *primary health care* as a term, but what does it actually mean?

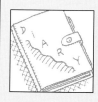

ACTIVITY 1
20 MINS
Write down in your diary what primary health care means to you.

Before we move on to look at who is involved in providing primary care and what these people do, we need to understand clearly the concept of primary health care. The simplest way to do this is to look at an expert's definition and analyse it. The definition of primary health care reproduced here is the one agreed by all the World Health Organisation member states at their international conference held in Alma–Ata (the then Soviet Union) during 1978:

'Primary health care is **essential** health care made universally **accessible** to individuals and families in the community by means **acceptable** to them, through their full **participation** and at a **cost** that the community and country can **afford**. It forms an integral part of the country's health system of which it is the **main focus**. It is the **first level** of contact of individuals, the family and the community with the national health system, bringing health care as **close as possible** to where people live and work'[1].

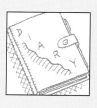

ACTIVITY 2
15-20 MINS
This definition is rather wordy. Re-read it and, with the help of the key words which appear in bold, break down the main objectives into a simple list.

Primary health care is a system for organising the planning and delivery of care to a given population. While every individual has particular health-care needs, it is easy to identify broad categories of people whose health needs at any one time are broadly similar.

The nursing review for Wales[2] identified the following client groups (which are not mutually exclusive) as needing primary health care services:
• Mothers and babies
• Adults
• The handicapped
• The temporarily injured or ill
• The long-term sick
• The frail elderly
• The dying.

Once client groups like those above have been identified, decisions have to be made about what type of care each group needs, how that care should be delivered, and who should deliver it. Obviously no one person could possibly have all the skills which would be needed to meet the demands of providing total care for everyone in the community. Over the past 20 years many GPs therefore have joined forces to set up group practices, often in purpose-built health centres, where they work alongside a number of other health workers, including nurses, midwives and administrators. Responsibility for patients is then shared, according to each worker's expertise, using a team approach — hence the primary health care team[3].

Primary health care agencies

Figure 1 shows six agencies which directly provide primary health care. The role of family and friends in providing informal primary care has also been included, as health problems are often resolved within the family with no recourse to outside agencies. For others, the informal carer is the main carer, while professional carers play a supportive role.

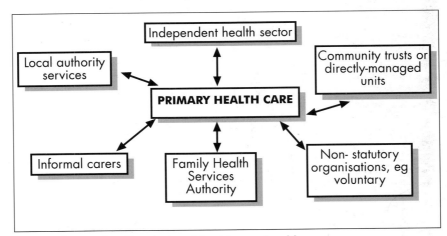

Fig 1. Those who directly provide primary health care

The 1990 NHS and Community Care Act gives these agencies new roles and responsibilities, and we will be exploring the implications of this for community nursing in Section 5 of this module.

ACTIVITY 3
2 HOURS

For your community profile copy out Figure 1 and insert the name of a contact you have made in four of the local equivalent services/organisations shown in Fig1.

If you made more than four contacts, include all of them. They will be a useful future resource for you.

Now make two lists: in the first, list the services for which the Family Health Services Authority (or its equivalent in your country) is responsible. In the second, list the health services that local government provides.

To obtain this information, either contact the relevant departments directly or look at your local community care plan which should contain a description of the services provided. You will be able to look at a copy of your local community care plan in your local library or social services department.

Add this information to your community profile

Community nurses' role in primary care

Having considered the different agencies which provide primary care, let us look more carefully at the roles of nurses in providing primary care. Figure 2 shows the different nurse roles involved. Some of these will work together as part of a health centre team, while others will work outside the immediate community team, but be closely linked to it.

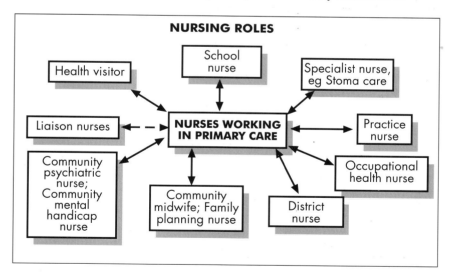

Fig 2. Community nurses in primary health care

The school nurse

School nurses aim to minimise all potential health problems which could impair a child's educational progress.

School nurses have increasingly moved away from a routine screening approach of 'bits of the body' and now undertake selective health interviews which capture the total health picture of the child. With this approach, health problems which the child identifies, such as the need for weight loss, can be dealt with using a special partnership programme, involving the child, the nurse and parents. Some school nurses run adolescent health advice sessions for senior school students; here teenagers can be sure of confidential support and advice on subjects as diverse as dealing with spots, exam pressures, or worries about sexuality and contraception.

One of the roles of the school nurse is that of health promotion (that is, promoting a healthy eating/lifestyle). However, this could create problems for the child if values and habits at home are different.

ACTIVITY 4
40 MINS
Make contact with a school nurse working near your home.

Ask her about her day-to-day timetable and how she promotes health both on an individual basis and in the classroom.

Ask her how she handles the potential conflict between the advice she gives to children and the values of their parents.

While much health education is carried out on a one-to-one basis very effectively, a growing number of school nurses are involved in the curriculum planning of their school's personal and social education programmes. Some nurses will actually teach, particularly sex education or about addictions, for example, while others may concentrate on linking health with other subjects in the curiculum, such as health statistics in mathematics or child care and good parenting in home economics.

School nurses have a special role with those children designated as having special needs under the Education Act 1978. These children receive regular assessments of need and the review of such children's progress can benefit greatly from the school nurse's contribution. The school nurse can observe the child at work and play in the school and bring together social and health information.

The health visitor
Health visitors are concerned with the total health of families, to whom they provide a continuing service offering advice, information and support. Health visitors work to promote health and prevent ill-health, rather than treating people. Preventing illness requires them to anticipate problems and to take appropriate action before difficulties arise. Their combination of health and social knowledge is invaluable for this role and influences their approach to care, which frequently involves liaison and close working with many other agencies.

Most health visitors' main client group is still mothers and pre-school children. The health visitor receives birth notifications from the hospital and visits every new baby (although frequently she will have worked with women antenatally). She then monitors that child's health and development until the child starts school, usually seeing mothers and young children in their own home or at clinic to work on promoting healthy development, and to assist women with the business of being new mothers.

Every authority has a child health surveillance programme and children undergo periodic developmental tests which the health visitors often conduct.

Health visitors work with many other groups in the community, such as elderly people who may need support in maintaining their health or adjusting to a loss of independence — they also provide advice for the carers.

Community health action programmes which help people address hazards to health in their environment are also part of the health visitor's remit. They may involve co-ordinating a campaign to lobby about condensation problems on a housing estate; setting up pensioners' food co-ops or enabling people who are isolated in the community, such as new mothers, to get together to support each other.

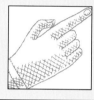

ACTIVITY 5
1 HOUR
Arrange to meet a health visitor and explore how she sees her role in the locality.

Another area in which many health visitors have responsibilities is abuse, whether of children or elderly people. The Children Act of 1989 has clarified the role of health professionals in child protection, and we will be discussing this in Section 5. In the same year, the British Geriatrics Society estimated that up to 500 000 elderly, highly dependent people could be at risk of physical or emotional abuse — often from their own families[4]. The Law Commission has recently called for local authorities to be given a statutory duty to investigate suspicious abuse of elderly people.

ACTIVITY 6
20 MINS
If you wish, during your meeting with the health visitor bring up the following issues:

Ask her to describe her responsibilities with regard to child protection.

Make a list of her points. If she also has an elderly caseload ask about her responsibilities with regard to the abuse of elderly people.

Make this part of your community profile.

Any clinic or health centre should keep a copy of the health authority's written guidelines with respect to child abuse. Only a few authorities have written guidelines with regard to abuse of elderly people.

The district nurse and district nursing team

The district nurse provides or organises skilled nursing care for sick and disabled people and their families, in their own homes. District nurses also work in health centres, providing care to ambulatory patients. As we saw in Section 1, the bulk of continuing home care is not given by professionals but by carers, so the district nurse spends considerable time assessing the carers' knowledge and ability to cope, and teaching

JOB DESCRIPTION

JOB TITLE: **District Nurse**
MINIMUM QUALIFICATIONS: **RN plus Certificate/Diploma in District Nursing**
ACCOUNTABLE TO: **Neighbourhood Nurse Manager**

JOB SUMMARY

1 To provide leadership, management and teaching skills to ensure the quality and continuity of nursing care.
2 To provide, promote and maintain a high standard of skilled nursing care to patients in their homes and in other environments.
3 To assess the needs of patients and carers and to be able to mobilise the appropriate resources.
4 To work as an effective member of the primary health care team in partnership with GPs and others.
5 To promote health and prevent illness.

DUTIES AND RESPONSIBILITIES

1 Assess the immediate and longer– term needs of patients and their carers.
2 Develop, implement and evaluate programmes of care.
3 Manage, co-ordinate and evaluate the work of the nursing team, ensuring the maintenance of clinical standards.
4 Offer support, advice and guidance to patients and their carers and be aware of, and utilise, appropriate resources and agencies.
5 Work as part of the primary health care team, liaising with colleagues and other statutory and voluntary agencies.
6 Promote good health practices whenever possible.
7 Keep up to date with clinical and professional developments.
8 Take part in the teaching and supervision of students within the community setting.
9 Assist with the organisation of cover for holidays, sickness and other leave of absence.
10 Keep accurate and contemporaneous records.
11 Encourage the use of research in the development of nursing practice.
12 Undertake forms of audit, revision and appropriate quality assurance activities.
13 Work within the guidelines of the Trust's policies and procedures.
14 To have responsibility for the health, safety and welfare of self and others in the working environment, to follow safe working practice, and to comply at all times with the Trust's health and safety policies and procedures.
15 To ensure confidentiality on all matters relating to patients and information obtained during the course of employment.
16 To undertake such other duties as may be reasonably required from time to time as are consistent with responsibility and scale of the post.
17 The post-holder will participate in the Trust's staff development and performance appraisal scheme.

techniques and skills, such as moving and lifting. They find themselves increasingly operating a programme of 'distance' management, delegating nursing care to their team of district enrolled nurses, community RGNs and auxiliaries, and reviewing outcomes.

A typical job description for a district nurse with Croydon Community Health Trust, reflecting the position in January 1993, is shown on the previous page.

Most district nursing services operate an extended service beyond the hours of 9am and 5pm. Some have 'twilight' care, although all-night provision is rare.

District nurses are skilled at managing and organising resources and plan their workload independently. They are able to select appropriately and mobilise a range of services for clients and have comprehensive knowledge about local voluntary and independent agencies from whom a range of help is available.

Following a referral, district nurses have to make careful judgements about how the resources available to the district nursing service are used, and this can lead to conflict. For example, not all GPs or social workers understand yet that the district nurse is likely to say 'no' to a request to carry out personal care tasks.

ACTIVITY 7
2 HOURS
Make arrangements to meet a district nurse. Ask her how she plans and assesses health care for the caseload she and her team are managing.

If you feel you can generalise from what she has said, indicate some points in your community profile about how district nurses plan and assess. Otherwise, make notes in your diary.

New areas of work for district nurses include a growing involvement with those suffering from AIDS and their partners, care for those who choose to die at home and care of sick children who are spending less time in hospital beds. In some areas, specialist community paediatric nurses are employed.

The practice nurse
On the next page is a typical job description from Enfield and Haringey FHSA reflecting the type of work carried out by practice nurses in January 1993[5]. Practice nurses are employed by general practitioners and their work has expanded rapidly over the past few years, from providing a limited range of clinical nursing care in the treatment room of the health centre, to running chronic disease clinics and health promotion sessions for the practice population

Practice nurses run their own 'surgeries', often alongside the GPs' own surgery sessions, where they receive referrals to carry out a wide range of activities, including injections, dressings, ear syringeing, teaching about drug therapy or assisting with minor surgery such as cryotherapy or cyst removal. The type of work they undertake is determined by the knowledge and competence of the nurse, the size and location of the practice, and the doctors' own interests.

One recent study found almost two-thirds of practice nurses carrying out breast and vaginal examinations and cervical smears, with a number also diagnosing, investigating and managing common ailments[6].

SPECIMEN JOB DESCRIPTION

POST:	**Practice nurse**
QUALIFICATIONS:	**Registered General Nurse; Practice Nurse Certificate; Family Planning ENB 901**
GRADE:	**G**
BASED AT:	**Surgery/Health Centre; Home visiting**
PROFESSIONALLY RELATES TO:	**FHSA Nurse Adviser; Local Nurse Manager**
ACCOUNTABLE TO:	**General Practitioners (you can specify one)**

JOB SUMMARY
To provide nursing services to patients of the practice including treatment, screeening, advice and teaching within the professional competence of the post-holder (extra training will be provided before new duties are undertaken). The post-holder will work in accordance with the UKCC Code of Conduct.

KEY RESPONSIBILITIES
Provides health screening and general nursing to the practice population and controls own caseload.

Develops, implements and evaluates health promotion clinics, including at least one specialist clinic like Diabetic, Asthma, Well Women, Menopouse.

Provides telephone advice on general health problems and some minor illness.

General nursing, which includes the assessment and management of minor ailments.

Responsible for the review and implementation of infection control measures.

Contributes to the development and review of practice protocols.

Develops and evaluates standards of nursing care.

Contributes to clinical audit.

Provides teaching and support to junior practice nurses and medical students.

OPTIONAL
Provides teaching for any community or general nurse students.

Provides and co-ordinates the elderly screening programme.

Contributes to research.

Manages a treatment room budget.

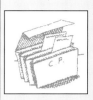

ACTIVITY 8
2 HOURS
Contact the practice nurse working for your own GP or at a health centre known to you. Ask her how her responsibilities have changed and developed over the past few years and what type of work she does.

Enter the outcome of this conversation in your community profile.

The family planning nurse

Family planning nurses rarely work full time but are generally community trained nurses who have taken a recognised course in family planning nursing and then work on a sessional basis. They are experts in contraception, with a knowledge of fertility issues and sexual health. Many family planning sessions are combined with well women checks. This branch of community nursing concentrates on detecting problems at an early stage and arranging for referral or treatment of, for example, suspected gynaecological conditions, cancer of the cervix and breast, or sexual dysfunction. Women can obtain information and advice about all aspects of their health from family planning nurses.

One of the targets in the government's strategy *The Health of the Nation*[7] is to reduce the rate of conceptions among the under 16s by at least 50% by the year 2000.

ACTIVITY 9
30 MINS
Make an appointment to visit the local manager of the family planning service and ask her to outline briefly the local strategy to achieve this target.

Make this Activity part of your community profile.

Did you find that the strategy included all the members of the primary health care team ? Were other agencies involved as well?

The occupational health nurse

People's health is closely related to the quality of the environment in which they are working. Occupational health nurses' efforts are directed toward ensuring the health and safety of workers. Nurses inspect work areas and are able to detect relationships between the physical and mental health of workers and particular stresses of their jobs.

Having looked at the roles played by the various nurse members of the primary health care team, we now turn to the team itself — to learn about what makes for effective teamwork.

What is teamwork?

It would be wrong to conclude this chapter without reflecting on the concept of teamwork. The principles of successful teamwork are as appropriate to your local primary health care team as to your local premier league football club, but in practice, genuine teamwork exists more as a concept than a reality[8]. The NHS and Community Care Act 1990 is now putting further demands on the primary health care team, in the emphasis on effective teamwork between different agencies.

Essential characteristics for good teamwork include:
1. Team members share a common purpose which binds them together and binds their action.
2. Each member of the team has a clear understanding of her own functions and recognises common interests.
3. The team works by pooling knowledge, skills and resources and all members share responsibility for outcome.
4. Respect for the individual skills of each member.
5. Each member communicates and at times negotiates her professional role with other members on an ongoing basis as services evolve[9].

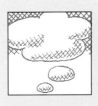

ACTIVITY 10
10MINS
Stop and reflect for a minute on the characteristics of teamwork identified above and ask yourself whether in your practice setting you work in a team of equals with a common goal of delivering quality care to patients.

Many teams work well together, but in some cases individual status, egos, bureaucratic organisation and differing philosophies get in the way of the goal. Team members in primary care need a clear understanding of their own and each other's role before they can share responsibility. But often there has been an assumption that if you put a collection of people in the same building, such as a health centre, they will automatically agree on a common task, share their knowledge and skills to meet that task and then share collective responsibility for the outcome.

Many district nurses and health visitors started to be 'attached' to general practices in the early 1960s and it was assumed that, almost by a process of osmosis, they would form teams alongside GPs without any support and professional education. However, as the joint working group on the primary health care team put it: 'Successful teamwork needs more than an agreement to work together'[10].

Blocks to effective teamwork
A report from the Audit Commission[11] has outlined the following barriers to effective working within primary health care teams. Different members of the team had:

1. Separate lines of control
2. Different payment systems leading to suspicion over motives (a reference to the fact that GPs are paid per item of service for some of their work)
3. Diverse objectives
4. Professional barriers
5. Perceived inequalities in status.

The report also noted the consequences:

•Rigidity within teams with members adhering to narrow definitions of their roles, preventing the creative and flexible responses required to meet the variety of human need presented. They are also likely to have lower morale. For nurses working under such circumstances efficient teamwork remains an elusive ideal.**•**

Happy teams

In primary care, most doctors and nurses enjoy working together and a lot of effort goes into making teamwork a happy and productive experience.

Teams which work well tend to do so by concentrating on planning the best outcomes of care for an individual/family with health needs and regularly reviewing whether those patients' needs are met.

There are a number of methods teams can adopt to improve their practice:
1. Make clear agreements about treatment, or the process of care. These agreements may be in the form of written protocols which all members of the team can sign and agree.
2. Hold regular, structured team meetings. As Hicks wrote about primary health teams' approach to communication: 'As much as I enjoy the coffee break, I have little faith in it as a managerial device'[12].
3. Provide opportunities for joint education on team building or opportunities to learn together about experimental approaches to care.

The wider team

Any assessment carried out by a nurse in the community will consider the total needs of the clients and often of their spouses, carers, parents or whole family. This might include their physical and mental health and may involve looking at their social situation (for example, financial and housing problems). Often, aspects of their emotional and sexual situation will be explored. The nurse determines jointly with the individual or with the family what their needs are and who can meet them. Rarely does one individual possess all the relevant skills needed and the community nurse practitioner judges which other agencies and personnel can contribute.

If, historically, communication within the primary health care team has been difficult, it is not surprising that communiction between personnel in other agencies such as local authorities has also been poor.

All too frequently joint working is a piecemeal affair, as the following exchange between a district nurse manager and a researcher highlights. The extract is from a study of the community care provided for 176 elderly people who are all visited by both health and social services practitioners.

•Interviewer: We asked the social workers [in your area] to tell us whether a district nurse was going to their clients. They often weren't sure and in about half the cases had it wrong.

DNM: Well, there is no reason why they shouldn't know. We leave notes in the patient's house and there is no reason why the social worker shouldn't see them.

Interviewer: Have you any idea how many of your patients are also social services clients?

DNM: None whatsoever'13.

One of the main aims of the NHS and Community Care Act of 1990 is to facilitate this essential communication between agencies, and we will explore this more fully in Section 5. Clearly there was a breakdown in communication in the example just cited, which could be alleviated by a forum in which the social worker and the community nurse could discuss matters of common interest, instead of leaving it to the client to tell both parties what is going on.

Such lack of communication has often been highlighted by inquiries into circumstances surrounding deaths from child abuse. It was reported, for example, between the health visitor and the social worker in the case of Jasmine Beckford, who died in 1985[14]:

'If only the two workers on this case had compared notes, they would have quickly discovered that they were being told different and contradictory stories (by the mother).'

The structure of care management as set out by the NHS and Community Care Act 1990 is aimed at improving inter-agency communication.

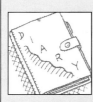

ACTIVITY 11
45 MINS
You now understand more about what primary care is and who is involved in providing it.

Below are three examples of people needing services. Consider who might be involved in planning, providing and monitoring the care they are likely to need, and make notes in your diary. (Look back at Figure 1 so that you know you have included all agencies engaged in primary care.)

1. A woman wanting shared antenatal care (that is, care is shared between her GP clinic and the hospital clinic) during her first pregnancy.

2. A 49-year-old woman who has recently given up her job to care for her elderly mother who has multiple sclerosis.

3. A baby attending for a combined measles, mumps and rubella immunisation (MMR).

Your list might have included the following:

1. Community midwives, GP, technicians, hospital clerical staff, practice receptionist, people running National Childbirth Trust antenatal classes, health visitor, hospital obstetric team, dentist.
2. The district nurse, GP, voluntary organisations (for example, Crossroads care attendant schemes, Age Concern), social worker, liaison nurse, occupational therapist, physiotherapist, neighbours, pharmacist at local chemist.
3. Health visitor, child health computer record clerk, Family Health Services Authority computer technician, GP or clinic medical officer, director of public health, receptionist, practice nurse.

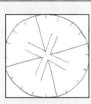

FOCUS
4-6 HOURS

Ask for details of the complete range of preventive health and other services which are available at your own health centre or GP surgery. All practices produce booklets or leaflets which provide you with information you might need about opening hours, waiting times, evening clinics, plus a profile of all the doctors, nurses and administrative staff employed there. Look through the information you have gathered when you get home and see if it includes details of:

- Child health clinics, immunisation and vaccination
- Screening clinics
- Well women or well men sessions
- Clinics for people with diabetes
- Family planning services
- Keep fit or dieting groups
- Giving-up-smoking groups/support
- Pregnancy testing
- Antenatal care
- The services of a counsellor or community psychiatric nurse
- Patient complaints mechanisms.

Did the waiting area and health promotion material on display pass your good practice test as well?

Contact your local FHSA (or the equivalent in your country) and ask for a copy of their minimum standards for premises. In what ways did your health centre or GP surgery relate to those standards?

From what you have collected, from your observations in the centre and from the reaction to your requests for information, assess how successful your local health team is. Record your opinion and discuss the ingredients of successful primary care teams at your next network meeting.

Enter your observations and the information you gather in your community profile.

3.Setting priorities in community health care

Section 1 looked at the identification of needs and Section 2 at the personnel who aim to tackle some of those needs. This Section will explore how the differing health needs lead comunity health services to set different priorities. On an individual level, too, community nurses, despite having similar job descriptions, may have different working styles.

However, not all the differences in provision between one part of the country and another are logical, planned differences. Spending on community health services varies considerably between health districts, with some spending twice as much per person as others![1] This would not be a bad thing if there were a close relationship between indicators of need (for example, the Jarman Index[2] which identified underprivileged areas, or the number of people over 75 — the main users of the district nursing service[1]) and the level of provision. However, there is little evidence to show a link between expenditure and demand.

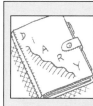

ACTIVITY 1
1 HOUR
Contact the information officer of your local health authority.

• Find out how much is spent per person on community health services in your authority.

• Contrast this with how much is spent in a neighbouring authority.

Make a note of any reasons which you believe would explain the variation.

There are no data available which will tell us whether twice the amount of spending will guarantee that patients will receive twice the quality of care. However, these sometimes considerable variations in spending do explain why some types of service and care available in one area of the country simply do not exist elsewhere.

Serving the needs of all

Well before any of the patients' charters were published, community nurses had been designing services which would ensure that everyone, including people with special needs, would be able to use any of the services (a requirement common to all of the charters). The 1980s saw a host of innovative schemes and new styles of working. An overview of some of the schemes aimed at preventive health care in pregnancy and early childhood has been documented[3].

Particular emphasis has been given to reaching clients who might find it difficult to use services, such as:
• Those not registered with a GP
• Travellers' families
• Housebound elderly
• Clients whose first language is not English.

Similarly, the community health services recognised that tackling issues such as prevention of coronary heart disease could not rely on conventional services, as many young and middle-aged people have minimal contact with the health services. Therefore, the health promotion activity has been taken to where people happen to be — the workplace, or a shopping centre.

ACTIVITY 2
1 HOUR
Make a list of any special service provisions in your locality, then choose one service from the list and find out:

• **Why the nurses in the community thought it was necessary to make special provision**
• **If they have evaluated how useful this service has been in meeting the need they identified**
• **If there is any information available about what the consumers think about this service.**

If no evaluation has been done from either the nurses' or the consumers' point of view, then approach some of the clients using the service and ask their opinion.

Include this information in your community profile.

Did your list include:
• Facilities which are open at unusual times, such as evening clinics?
• Clinics in unusual places, such as caravans, church halls or rooms in housing estates?
• Facilities where the public could walk in or walk by and get information, such as 'health information desks' at clinics or market stalls?
• Special outreach workers who work with groups such as drug abusers or prostitutes?
• Groups of health workers who had a team approach to a specific problem?
• Instances where community nursing staff worked alongside volunteers or self-help groups, or indeed took a back-seat supportive role to a self-help group?
• New types of documentation developed to assist care (for example, client-held records or special information sheets)?

Evaluating the new ways of working

One of the major problems faced by community staff when provider units give the go-ahead for the provision of new types of community health care is that the unit may fail to guarantee long-term funding.

The only weapon that community nursing staff have at their disposal in their effort to maintain a new service is facts and figures about the extent of the need and facts and figures about their own effectiveness in meeting that need. An example of this would be the way health visitors working with homeless families have participated in research on the health needs of their clients which indicates that these clients are facing an above average incidence of:
• Infectious disease (from diarrhoea to TB)
• Accidents
• Mental health problems
• Development/behavioural problems in children
• Problems of pregnancy (for example, low birth-weight babies)
• Increased hospital admission or attendances[4].

Measuring the effectiveness of community nursing staff in this situation is very difficult as the number of homeless families is continuing to grow. However, health visitors can indicate the percentage of homeless families known to be in an area that they have made contact with and the number of health problems they have detected, treated or referred.

ACTIVITY 3
2 HOURS
Find out from your FHSA/DHA/community health council (or the equivalent in your country)/ the members of the community nursing team you have met, if there has been any attempt to evaluate any aspect of community nursing provision in your area formally (for example, by means of a consumer survey). If not, arrange to visit your local community health council and discuss the different types of complaints which arise about community services.

Note down your findings in your community profile.

Setting priorities

A traditional view of nursing in the community would see nurses as visiting individual clients at home. However, practitioners can also be working with:
• Individual clients
• Families
• Groups of clients with similar needs
• Groups of families with similar needs
• People in a specified geographical area (for example, a housing estate)
• The community as a whole.

Alternatively, practitioners may be participating in a regionally or nationally co-ordinated health promotion activity[5] such as the 'Heartbeat Wales' programme aimed at preventing heart disease in the principality.

All the different styles of work reflect an attempt to make a limited resource (that is, the community nursing service) more effective in tackling health needs and in preventing ill-health by working in the most appropriate way for the needs of each group.

In the same way that a service can be planned in order to make it more available to clients with particular health needs, so individual practitioners can look at their own caseload in the light of the research which indicates that some clients might be more at risk of ill-health than others, and set priorities accordingly.

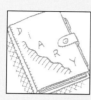

ACTIVITY 4
15-30 MINS
Ask any member of the community nursing team that you are in contact with, which client they visit most often.

Explore the reasons for the frequency of visits.

Are they determined by the client's clinical condition (or in the case of visiting a healthy child, by the age of the child) or is the pattern of visiting determined by social or other factors?

Note your thoughts in your diary.

Setting priorities is always a matter of professional judgement. Practitioners often worry that time spent with one client or a group of clients may have a detrimental effect on others. This can even be a problem within one household! Consider the following examples:

1. An elderly relative is cared for by another family member. Sometimes what is best for the elderly person has a detrimental effect on the carer. How does the district nurse best support the family?

2. A health visitor visiting a family where a child has been abused may feel torn that a decision made in the interests of the child may have a devastating effect on the mother or father. The 1989 Children Act is clear that the child's needs are paramount, but is the child's health an entirely separate entity from the parents' health? How does the health visitor best support the family?

ACTIVITY 5
10 MINS
Both the situations described above are ethical dilemmas. There is no right or wrong answer. Try to describe what your feelings would be in both instances.

Jot down your findings in your diary.

Where do you put the emphasis?
Setting priorities within a caseload means a lot more than which clients to visit most often. It might mean taking an entirely different approach, such as deciding to see clients in a group setting. For example, it might be easier to meet the needs of carers by helping to set up a carers' group, where the mutual support that carers can give each other might be more effective than that offered by the health professional.

ACTIVITY 6
1 HOUR
Arrange to visit a self-help group that exists in your area or arrange to speak to the group facilitator/co-ordinator. Find out why it was set up and how. What input does it have, if any, from professional nursing staff? Is the work of the group viewed positively or negatively by community nursing staff?

Make a note of your findings in your community profile.

Setting priorities also extends to what topics you might choose to discuss with clients.

Consider the following statement from a co-ordinator for a special team of health visitors who visit homeless families housed in 140 hotels in Central London[6]:

'Because we were prepared to accept that the primary need was for social security and housing advice, access to GPs and the use of a drop-in centre for company and cooking facilities, mothers were then prepared to accept our own particular advisory role on health issues such as nutrition and child behaviour'.

Knowledge about social security benefits is often seen as a social worker's job. However, the link between income and health is undisputed, so meeting health needs means identifying individuals and families who may be eligible for benefit. Nurses do not need to be expert in this field, but it is clear that if they do not identify people who may be eligible, claims might not be made. Nurses should also be aware of where their clients might seek expert advice if required.

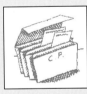

ACTIVITY 7
2 HOURS
Go to your local DSS office and collect the leaflets which describe social security benefits which are available for a particular client group (for example, disabled people or single parents). Critically examine the material.

- Is it written in an easy-to-understand fashion?
- Are the criteria for who is eligible for benefit made clear?
- Is there somewhere for clients to be referred for further advice if they have difficulty with benefits?
- Are the leaflets available in other community languages?
- Is the print big enough for those with a visual impairment?

Tailoring advice to individual circumstances
Awareness of people's financial circumstances is vital when offering health promotion advice. A report, *Shopping for Food*, published by the Welsh Consumer Council[7], found that healthy eating meant spending more on food. For example, they found wholemeal bread cost as much as 10p a loaf more than sliced white bread and that lean minced beef

could cost up to 62p per lb more than ordinary minced beef. It was also found that shoppers could save up to 10% by shopping in large supermarkets, but many people in rural areas have access to only a small local shop.

ACTIVITY 8
1 HOUR

Select four staple items such as tea, bread, fruit, rice and contrast prices in a small local shop with the nearest large supermarket. Assess how accessible the supermarket is to people with disabilities, and non-car owners.

Record your findings in your community profile.

Awareness of cultural differences is also important.

ACTIVITY 9
1 HOUR

Contact your local health promotion department and ask to look at their range of health promotion literature on healthy eating.

• Consider whether this literature would be suitable for all of the groups in your local community.

If it is not suitable, make some notes in your diary as to how you think it could be revised to suit their needs.

It must be borne in mind that knowledge of the client's circumstance does not always make it easy to give advice or offer support. For example, health visitors conscious of the safety hazards that many children face in the home do not find it easy to advise parents on purchase of safety equipment when they know that a family has financial problems. Consider the following statement from a study carried out by Pamela Laidman[8] for the Child Accident Prevention Trust:

'The health visitors also reported that to certain clients some accident risks could not be mentioned, even when they were present, due to the risk it may place upon their relationship with the client. This was most common when to mention the hazard the health visitor may be seen as critical of the client. Also, when the safety advice had been given several times before unsuccessfully, the health visitors found they had to stop or risk their relationship with the client.'

Sometimes the reality of setting priorities is that some health needs must be deliberately overlooked in order for practitioners and clients to work together on addressing other health needs.

Protocols — a way of increasing effectiveness

Contradictory advice and lack of continuity can undermine nursing care in any setting. In the community this can pose special problems as clients can see different members of the primary health care team in a variety of settings.

To this end, many primary health care teams have developed protocols – guidelines which help clarify roles and responsibilities and ensure that the best practice is consistently followed. Developments in this field have covered conditions such as hypertension, diabetes and asthma[1], as well as areas such as advice given to mothers about breast-feeding. In order to offer a truly 'seamless service', some protocols extend beyond the primary health care team and include hospital services.

ACTIVITY 10
30 MINS
Ask at your local health centre or surgery whether they have designed any protocols for practice.

Ask any member of the primary health care team covered by the protocol what are its benefits (or problems!)

If possible, take a photocopy of the document and include it in your community profile.

Inter-agency working

Communication and co-ordination between different services in the community has always been difficult. The 1990s will see renewed efforts to improve systematically this aspect of care. The Children Act 1989, implemented in October 1991, requires the setting up of area child protection committees to address the problem of co-ordination in the field of child protection. The NHS and Community Care Act 1990 demands a process of care management which should also improve communication between agencies.

ACTIVITY 11
2 HOURS
Contact a community nurse manager and arrange to be an observer at a multidisciplinary meeting between the community health services and social services.

Record your observations in your community profile.

In your opinion, did the participants at the meeting have a clear understanding of each other's role or did they frequently seek clarification? Were there many points of conflict or controversy? Did the meeting keep clients' needs as the main focus of the agenda?

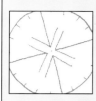

FOCUS
1 HOUR

The Focus Activity for this Section asks you to look at what strategy or approach the community health services in your locality have taken to address a particular problem. Health needs are never static. New problems constantly arise, such as the increased incidence of HIV/AIDS, or osteoporosis.

- Ask a community health service manager, or the department of public health of your health authority or board, about any new initiative to tackle a health problem that they have taken this year.

OR

- Ask what new steps the above agencies are taking to reach one of the targets set out in the government's *Health of the Nation* report[9]. A copy of the full report should be available in your college library.

- List the community personnel involved
- Find out how the initiative involves other agencies
- Find out whether the public are involved in the initiative
- Think about whether you observed any aspect of this new work while on your placement. If you did, write down your thoughts about it.

Note down your own ideas of how community practice could be developed to meet the problem or target you select.

4.Delivering and planning home care

Throughout this Section we will be inviting you to reflect on how your own community experience is similar to or different from what we describe.

The case study used here will illustrate many of the factors involved in delivering and planning home care. It is not intended to be a 'perfect' example of nursing care. Indeed, space does not permit us to include many of the details of the care given. Rather, it is hoped that it will act as a stimulus to your thoughts and discussions about nursing in the community.

Before we go any further, let's introduce the presenting problem in the case study.

District nurse Ann Wilson had just finished her clinic at the health centre when Dr Anderson, one of the GPs she worked with, put his head round the door and said:

'Ann, could you just pop by and see a Mrs Judy Betts of 76 Langemere Avenue. She's got a young family and is keen to look after her mother who is terminally ill with breast cancer. I told her that it was a bit unrealistic but she seems determined to have a try. See what you think.'

Ann just had time to scribble down the address before Dr Anderson was heading out of the door clutching his list of home visits.

Knowing the health visitor attached to the practice had only recently arrived and did not yet know the family, Ann left a note to say she was visiting Mrs Betts.

Referrals

In a hospital setting, patients are either booked admissions or emergency admissions. The referral to Ann Wilson was one of many ways that a referral may come to nurses working in the community. Referrals may also come from:

- The antenatal clinic (midwife)
- Health visitors (who have been notified about new births)
- GPs
- Clients (they contact the nurse directly)
- Hospital nurses, including liaison nurses
- Social services departments
- Other local authority departments (for example, housing department)
- Neighbours/friends
- School teachers
- Education welfare officers
- Voluntary agencies
- The police
- Residential homes
- Nursing homes.

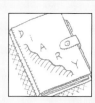

ACTIVITY 1
1 HOUR
All nursing records should indicate the source of referral. Arrange to look at six sets of case notes of a community nurse and make a note of the source of referral, and the information supplied to the community nurse on referral.

Discuss with the nurse how adequate the quality of the referral information was.

From the long list of the sources of referral you might suspect that community nursing caseloads could grow like Topsy. This does happen! Examples of this would be where a new housing estate is built and a large number of young families move in, or when the main employer in a town closes down.

When Ann Wilson checked her diary she realised that she had very little time available that day. She decided that a short hurried visit would not be appropriate as Mrs Betts might be conscious of the limited time and could feel disinclined to begin to explain a complicated situation and merely insist 'I'm coping fine!'. Ann therefore decided to visit the next day, allowing herself an hour, but she was unable to telephone Judy Betts beforehand because she got caught up in other work. However, when she explained on the doorstep that Dr Anderson had asked her to call, Judy Betts cordially invited her in.

As soon as she entered the room Ann realised that Judy Betts had already put quite a lot of effort into planning her mother's care. The house had a through lounge, one end of which seemed normally to function as a dining room. The dining table was now pushed against the wall and acted as a surface for her mother's belongings and a small divan bed with a mountain of pillows had been moved into that end of the room. Her mother was sitting in an easy chair watching TV in the other part of the room. Although this part of the room had no furniture in it apart from the easy chairs and the TV, brightly coloured interlocking storage boxes of toys filled the corners.

The children, Emma (three years) and Joy (15 months), had been in the garden when Ann arrived but came in to investigate at the little door which led from the lounge to the garden. They were both warmly wrapped against the November air. As Mrs Betts opened the door Joy pulled herself into the room and made a dive for her mother's legs. Emma was more circumspect and watched the stranger from the door.

In the exchange that followed Ann Wilson learnt that Mrs Betts' mother — who was called Lucy Maycroft — had been living in her own council flat 50 miles away, until six days ago. Mrs Maycroft felt rather weak but was able to do most things for herself. Her appetite was 'not brilliant' but she did enjoy some foods. She mentioned a small 'sore' on her breast which was 'becoming a bit more troublesome'. She slept downstairs at night and took a nap in the day when the baby had her sleep. She explained that Dr Anderson had prescribed dihydrocodeine 30mg for night-time and she took paracetamol during the day. He had also prescribed something for ▶

her bowels, but she wondered whether this was necessary as she was eating a little more and getting about a bit. Ann reassured her that it was appropriate to prescribe an aperient when taking a drug which constipates.

Ann also learnt that Mr Jack Betts worked as a maintenance engineer at a local factory. He worked overtime fairly regularly as this helped with mortgage repayments, which were a 'bit of a struggle' since Mrs Betts had given up her part-time job before Joy was born. As Mrs Betts talked, Ann was mentally listing the multiple demands made on Mrs Betts: a husband coming home late and probably hungry, two young children, a sick mother... However, Mrs Betts was singularly uncomplaining and the only specific difficulty that she mentioned was that Emma had not been able to get a place in the local nursery school and this meant that 'Emma really needs entertaining, especially in the afternoons'.

Initial assessment

After the referral, the first contact with the client becomes a very important occasion for gathering facts, interpreting feelings and beginning to get some sort of sense of what the situation comprises. The initial assessment also moves from impressions to planning.

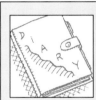

ACTIVITY 2
10 MINS
Put yourself in Ann Wilson's place and try to answer the following questions based on the observations she made during the initial assessment:

- Who do you think is the client in this scenario?
- Can you meet all the demands of everyone involved?
- If not, how can you prioritise them in your role as a community nurse?

Make notes in your diary.

The latter part of Ann Wilson's assessment visit gave her an opportunity to speak to Mrs Maycroft alone. Ann explained that the 'sore' was probably a fungating ulcer which would require a dressing. Mrs Maycroft was happy for Ann to examine the ulcer and made her way slowly and rather stiffly to the divan bed. Mrs Betts meanwhile took the children into the garden. When Ann examined Mrs Maycroft's left breast, she found it was a solid tumour mass with a fungating ulcer to the left of the nipple. The ulcer was malodorous and would clearly require regular dressing, probably with a dressing containing charcoal which would reduce the odour. In fact, the frequency of dressing changes would be one of the determining factors in the pattern of visiting Mrs Maycroft would require. Ann made a mental note to let Dr Anderson know about her observations because they might indicate an aerobic infection was present which would need treatment.

Mrs Maycroft took this opportunity to explain to Ann that she had first discovered a lump in her breast three years ago but had been reluctant to seek treatment. Eventually her daughter had persuaded her to see the doctor when the ulcer appeared and her arm became swollen. She explained that she had refused any radical treatment. 'I'm 67; I know it's not as old as some but I'm just going to take the future little by little.'

Mrs Maycroft also seized this moment of privacy to explain that she slept rather fitfully and always needed to use the toilet at night. She said that her daughter invariably heard her slow progress on the stairs and came out to help. She felt that this tired her daughter and added 'I doubt that Jack [Mr Betts] is too pleased either'. Ann explained that a commode could be provided and Mrs Maycroft was more than happy to use one — clearly she had been quite anxious about this.

This discussion about fitful sleep seemed to lead quite naturally to a more in-depth discussion of how Mrs Maycroft viewed her illness and her fears about death. Uncontrollable pain was obviously something which worried her and so Ann was able to explain about symptom control at home.

Assessment and planning are never distinct categories and Ann was already formulating a list of things to be done.

ACTIVITY 3
30 MINS
Ask a member of the community nursing team how practitioners in community nursing and social services communicate with one another about client care. List the methods in your diary.

You might have considered: contact by letter, telephone, computer, fax, face-to-face meetings, joint liaison meetings, case conferences, shared client records or joint care plans.

In our case study, Ann Wilson undertook the initial assessment, having received a GP referral. Ann then co-ordinated a network of services and specialist advice to meet the family's needs, as shown below in Figure 1.

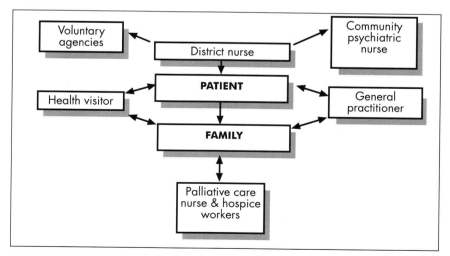

Fig 1. Primary care support for a dying patient

The figure shows the general practitioner, district nurse and health visitor as primary assessors. In this case Ann, the district nurse, is the care co-ordinator.

As Ann drove away from her assessment visit she reflected that what had struck her most about this family was their quiet determination that Mrs Maycroft's remaining time should be spent with her loved ones as comfortably as possible. She felt that her role and that of her colleagues was to give them support in that aim. Her first thought was to contact Julia Robb of the palliative care team. She knew that Julia was visiting another client in the locality tomorrow and decided to see if she could meet her at the health centre, together with Rebecca Johns, the health visitor attached to Dr Anderson's practice.

Nurse specialists in the community

The number of people choosing to die at home is growing and, in one study, community-based support teams were found to be more acceptable to dying people and their families than services from hospital doctors and nurses[1]. Palliative care teams have developed over the past decade to provide extra help and support for these patients, in co-operation with nurses and doctors already involved in their care[2].

ACTIVITY 4
5 MINS
Ask yourself why we need specialist nurses for dying people when every district nurse or health visitor has the skills to care for terminally ill people and their families.

Note down your thoughts in your diary.

The key aims of a nurse specialist in palliative care are to[1]:
• Control symptoms
• Give support and advice to patients, carers and professionals
• Co-ordinate care
• Meet practical needs
• Provide comprehensive, continuing assessments
• Provide education and bereavement support.

The meeting with specialist nurse Julia Robb and health visitor Rebecca Johns proved to be very useful. A whole aspect of care which Ann had not considered at the assessment visit was discussed, namely the reaction of the children to their sick grandmother and their possible reactions to her eventual death.

The health visitor was also able to explain that the shortage of nursery school places was a result of difficulties in recruiting teachers. She had heard, however, that a teacher returning after a career break might be recruited.

Time flew by and Ann realised that this meeting must have some clear outcome. It was decided that Ann would be the key worker with this family. Julia Robb would make a joint visit with her to the family. Rebecca Johns would investigate the nursery situation and would then visit the family.

Ann, in conjunction with her district nurse colleague, would plan frequency of visits, taking into account dressing changes, any assistance with physical care and emotional aspects. Their aim was to ensure there were no gaps in care and no duplication either. Ann told Julia that on her assessment visit she had not discussed the special rule element of the Attendance Allowance with Mrs Betts. A person caring for a terminally ill dependant with a prognosis of no more than six months is entitled to extra benefits. This would help with heating costs or special food. Julia agreed to leave an information pack at the health centre for Ann to take to the family.

For the generic nurse in the community, the specialists are used as a resource. Their expertise can be tapped into, perhaps a joint visit can be planned, and together an agreed programme of care can be co-ordinated which the community nurse will organise.

ACTIVITY 5
10 MINS
What is your experience of drawing on the skills of the specialist nurse system in your own practice setting? What do you find are its strengths and drawbacks?

Compare your thoughts with those of a community nurse with whom you have contact.

Nurse specialists work across the divide of acute and community care and act as a 'bridge'. They are able to bring new developments out to community nurse practitioners and the reverse is also true.

Specialists always aim to work in tandem with their community nurse colleagues so that 'seamless' care is achieved (for example, as you will see later, Ann Wilson visited the hospice and then participated in Mrs Maycroft's care).

Systematic care planning for community nursing practice

Recording what you plan to do, how you intend to do it and then measuring how successful you were in achieving your goals underpins all nursing practice. Without accurate, relevant, up-to-date and planned records, community nurses' accountability would be called into question. Indeed, the very first time a health visitor was called to account by the UKCC it was over concerns about her record-keeping.

Until recently few, if any, colleagues would refer to a school nurse's or health visitor's client records — including the client. There is a move within the profession to shift this balance of power; for example, a national parent-held child health record is now widely available in which all health professionals will record their findings. The Bristol Child Development Project has designed a programme of health visiting which actively encourages client participation and empowers mothers – particularly in impoverished communities — to control the recording process[3].

Client-held records have also been introduced by practitioners working with the homeless. Initially this was expedient, owing to the high levels of mobility among these users, but the positive spin-offs which accrued through the growth of mutual trust have led many health visitors to apply the principle of 'open' recording to their total caseload[4].

Some health visitors have felt dogged by a 'health by stealth' image or a social policing tag and believe that their claims to be health advocates for local communities are meaningless if the clients are excluded from the process of health visiting. They have found that sharing the means of recording with clients has a number of benefits.

District nurses have always placed their care plan in the patient's hands. This way, other clinical staff can easily access the home-based patient records and add to them. In theory this sounds excellent practice, demonstrating how nurses can empower patients by sharing all information and enabling the wider primary care team to communicate easily with one another. In practice, the district nursing record is often an incomplete picture, with scant reporting of treatment and care planned and a heavy orientation towards tasks performed. The 'real' records are kept back at base. It has been argued that such an approach to care planning does a disservice to the holistic nursing care which a skilled district nurse would be delivering or monitoring[5].

Little systematic research has been undertaken of district nursing records and the measurement of outcomes, but the introduction of tools to assess and evaluate the quality of nursing care has been an encouraging move. As anyone is now able to consult records held on them by a health professional there is likely to be greater attention paid by nurses to how they approach recording[6].

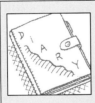

ACTIVITY 6
15 MINS
Think back to when you started training as an enrolled nurse and reflect on how patients participated in their own health assessment, history-taking or contributed to care planning records, chart-keeping, and so on. Do you think this situation has changed?

If you consider that patients are more active today in setting goals and evaluating their care jointly with nurses or other health professionals, write down in your diary what you think has contributed to this change.

You might have included:
1. Models of nursing care which are rooted in the use of a systematic, goal-oriented approach to recording.
2. Patient's charter rights and standards which promote the sharing of information with users.
3. Professional changes, such as the introduction of primary nursing with more explicit personal and professional accountability for care.
4. The Data Protection Act which gives patients rights to access their health records.

Quantifying nursing in the community

> At the end of the week, as Ann looked at her statistical returns for that week, she spent a moment reflecting on how initial contacts with families can be time-consuming — her visit, the lunch-time meeting, not to mention telephone calls! It had taken 20 minutes to get through to the hospital switchboard to contact the palliative care team! Roll on the new switchboard.

Community nurses have always been required to return certain basic information about workload for local and national statistical purposes, but until recently the data collected on community nursing activity were fairly meaningless, trawling 'numbers of homes visited' or 'numbers of various clients seen in the previous month'.

One shrewd observer of primary health care commented that collecting data in this case was, 'Interesting but it is a bit like counting the rivets in the *Queen Mary*, which would tell us nothing about how well the ship functions'[7]. Clearly, monitoring and evaluating community nursing practice should indicate what has been achieved and how the service could provide more effective care.

In 1984 this was partially addressed when the Körner committee wrote its report on community information requirements[8], and recognised that you could not helpfully measure health visiting, for example, just by counting people. This report attempted to include data collection on the full range of activities engaged in by nurses in the community. You will hear people talk about 'Körner minimum data sets' and they are referring to the information that every health authority has had to collect on community nursing workload since April 1988. These data do not, however, include the large amount of sensitive social and community health knowledge from community health profiles which community nurses use to prioritise the need for their skills in their own local area.

Computers in the community

Microcomputing facilities, because of their portability, are proving attractive to community nurses. These flexible systems can provide detailed information on each nurse, her clients, associated workload, record maintenance and systematic care planning. The use of fax machines has improved hospital-community liaison greatly in recent years.

In the past few years a range of hand-held terminals has been designed. These store information on micro-cassettes for processing by a centrally-based computer. The advantage to practitioners is that they can carry a terminal on their visits, tap in the required data and feed this back to the centre once a day. They can also generate a lot of useful data quickly, which helps in giving an overview of who is providing what to whom. There are no fully integrated community and hospital systems yet, but the day is not far off when a carefully arranged hospital discharge plan could be delivered to the community nurse without delay, while her community nursing assessment could be accessed by ward nurses on admission, so avoiding the need for duplication of effort.

Immunisation and vaccination

When Rebecca Johns telephoned Judy Betts to arrange a home visit, the immediate response was, 'You just reminded me! Joy's MMR injection was due two weeks ago. It completely slipped my mind with Mum arriving'. As a result Rebecca arranged to see Mrs Betts and the children after the child health clinic. Mrs Betts arranged for a neighbour to stay with her mother.

MMR, referred to in the case study, is a combined measles/mumps/rubella vaccine, now given to children at between 12 and 18 months.

The management of local child immunisation and vaccination programmes is one of the health visitor's key roles. Health visitors spend a lot of time ensuring parents receive appropriate advice and education about the importance of immunisation programmes[9].

The Department of Health sets child immunisation attainment targets for all health authorities and GPs. For example, by 1995, 95% of all children should have been immunised. This target-setting has improved uptake in many areas, though often this has been due to clearing up the way the data on immunisations are recorded, rather than the giving of more injections. Some districts have already surpassed the 95% target[10].

In North America, parents have to give exceptional reasons for not immunising their children before entry to school and school entry can be barred if immunisation is incomplete. As a consequence uptake is extremely high, and the incidence of measles and rubella low. Parents who do not take on this responsibility are seen as anti-social, because they endanger other children in the community. Do you think we should encourage such measures and foster these attitudes in Britain?

ACTIVITY 7
10 MINS
Look at the health promotion literature on MMR or *Haemophilus influenzae* Type B (HIB) which is available at your local health centre/clinic, and read it carefully.

When you have done this, ask the health visitor, GP or practice nurse what the uptake is in their area and note down the answer in your community profile.

There are still districts in Britain which achieve only 60-70% uptake of measles immunisation. What reasons might account for this?

ACTIVITY 8
20 MINS
When you are next together with your peer group, compare your findings on Activity 7. Discuss together what reasons parents might have for not immunising their children and highlight the measures your group would introduce to change their approach. Note down in your diary the views expressed.

Here are some of the points you might have considered:
- A belief that 'measles isn't too bad — she'll get it when it goes round'
- Clinics are held at inconvenient times (such as when the mother is at work) and immunisation is not always available at the GP's surgery
- Fear of side-effects
- Parents confused about arguments for and against immunisation and the result is to opt out
- If the professionals' own knowledge about immunisation is deficient in any way, patients may be reluctant to act on their advice
- Parents not aware of the importance of immunisation programmes to the community's health
- The child had already suffered from measles, leading parents to think an injection was no longer needed.

Caring for the carers

When Rebecca met Judy Betts after the clinic she explained that there was now a strong possibility that the local nursery would be able to offer Emma a place after Christmas. Mrs Betts was very pleased. However, as Rebecca went on to explain that the school would expect her (or her husband) to spend some time at the school initially to help settle Emma, Judy Betts looked rather worried. She explained that she wouldn't be happy to leave her mother for any length of time and neighbours could not be expected to help out on a regular basis. 'On the other hand, Emma really needs to go', she mused. She went on to reflect how Emma had had a rather difficult time. Initially Emma had been pleased when her 'Nana' came to stay, but Mrs Betts now sensed that the child felt squeezed out by the urgent demands of a 15-month-old and a sick grandmother.

During the rest of the interview Judy Betts felt free to express some rather conflicting emotions. She felt confident that caring for her mother at home was the right thing to do; on the other hand she felt guilty that the children might suffer. 'Not to mention Jack. I really haven't the energy to talk to him in the evenings, so he sometimes goes out and has a bit too much to drink because he feels left out.' She also mentioned that her husband was concerned about the fact that their heating bills were bound to rise.

Rebecca did a great deal of listening during this interview. There was no ready answer to these conflicting demands on Mrs Betts. However, she did steer the conversation gently towards the possibility of Mrs Betts' mother being able to be alone for the short periods that Emma would initially attend the nursery – maybe one-and-a-half hours or so.

Rebecca explained to Mrs Betts that the family was eligible to apply for a Macmillan Grant to cover the cost of extra heating. Mrs Betts was happy for Rebecca to pursue this and Rebecca made a note to contact Julia – specialist nurses are often more familiar with the voluntary-aided support available in their field.

During the above interview the health visitor had been acutely aware of some of the clues Mrs Betts had been giving about the impact her caring role had been having on her family as a whole.

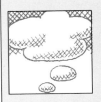

ACTIVITY 9
2-3 MINS
Think about Mrs Betts' casual remarks about not having sufficient 'energy' for her husband and about his drinking habits.

They could be straightforward factual statements. But do you think they could be indicative of other concerns Mrs Betts might have?

Did you consider how the family situation could lead to marital tension? Or the effect of night-time disturbance on a married couple's relationship and the general stress it could cause?

Although the health visitor encouraged Mrs Betts to develop the point, Mrs Betts had not taken the opportunity. However, receptiveness to these cues is an essential part of the community nursing role, as it gives clients 'permission' to raise the issue at a subsequent visit. Rebecca Johns could certainly remember instances when she had needed the support of her community psychiatric nurse colleagues in a similar situation, and mentally made a note to confer with them about possible support for Mr Betts once the family's current emotional crisis had passed. His wife's strain was increased by his withdrawal during this difficult period, but this situation needed to be rebuilt slowly.

Risk-taking: an ethical dilemma

You will note from the interview between Rebecca Johns and Judy Betts that the health visitor was 'encouraging' Mrs Betts to leave her mother for short periods. Helping clients make difficult choices is part of the community nurse's skill.

For example, maintaining a safe environment is a priority of hospital care. However, you will visit homes in the community which are 'unsafe', and see situations which are distinctly 'risky' by hospital standards (for example, clients with varying degrees of confusion living alone).

Nurses working in the community are always interested in their clients' safety, but they must respect their wishes and in particular their wish to be independent. Sometimes the client's neighbours disagree and insist that the nurse 'sorts out the situation'.

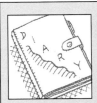

ACTIVITY 10
10 MINS
Try to put yourself in the shoes of a nurse working in the community who meets a neighbour who insists that an elderly, mildly confused client should be in a home. The elderly client has said that she would 'rather be dead than in a home'.

What would you say? How would you feel? What issues do you think are involved here?

Record your thoughts in your diary.

Relieving pressures on carers

Six million people are cared for at home by relatives and most of this burden is taken on by women. You will learn more about carers, in terms of government planning and social policy, in Section 5. We would like to think here about how you assess the needs of carers as an extension of your nursing actions for their dependants. All nurses come into contact with carers, whether they look after handicapped children, frail elderly, disabled or mentally ill people. Yet carers — who need information about local services they can tap into and availability of financial benefits, as well as practical tips about caring — often go unheard by professionals.

Carers' support groups

To meet this need, district nurses and health visitors are increasingly setting up and participating in carers' support groups, providing the chance for the carer to relax and attend the group safe in the knowledge that a volunteer helper is 'sitting' with their dependant.

Although the impetus for setting up a carers' group often emanates from the practical need for information, a great deal of the discussion at such groups focuses on the *emotional* and *psychological* impact of caring.

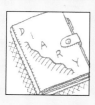

ACTIVITY 11
2-3 MINS
List as many factors as you can think of which would contribute to the mental stress of caring.

Some of the issues which carers mention include:
- The great sense of loss involved in watching the person they love deteriorate physically or mentally (carers of those with mental illness such as dementia may say: 'The person I knew died some time ago')
- The sensation of being trapped (owing to multiple demands, financial constraints, guilt feelings, and so on)
- The feeling of responsibility being entirely on the carer's shoulders
- The fact that the relationship between the carer and dependant had never been a good one—yet now they were being 'forced' on each other.

Nurses often teach carers basic nursing skills during sessions; for example, as experts in ways to move and handle safely, they can pass on this knowledge, or they will work with the community physiotherapist. One survey found that over one-third of carers admitted to having developed back pains[11].

ACTIVITY 12
60-90 MINS
Find out what respite care facilities are available for carers locally and list these in your community profile. Crossroads Care schemes, Help the Aged or Age Concern branches, MIND or your local community health council or a volunteer carer relief scheme attached to the local hospice

cont...

...cont

are among the organisations which can help you. Other questions to ask as part of this exercise are:

- What categories of people are admitted?
- Is there a waiting list?
- How frequently can carers obtain respite care and for how long?
- Who controls admission? Do community nurses have admitting rights?
- Do volunteer bureaux provide sitting services which allow carers short respite to shop or visit the cinema?
- Is there a charge?

Drawing on the information you have gathered, do you think carers in your area get a good deal, or is there a pool of unmet need? Support your judgement by drawing on the evidence you have gathered and share your written opinion with your support group.

Carers also suffer financially — Mr Betts worried about the increased heating bills; for other families, loss of earnings over the years reduces them to poverty. While community nurse practitioners would not he expected to understand all the details of the different benefits which are available, they frequently assist clients in making claims and actively liaise with agencies such as the Citizens' Advice Bureau or local social services department. Carers have precious little free time and find it very difficult to establish what they are entitled to, so the nurse's role, hooking people into benefits, is important.

Extra money is available for carers whose total income is low. They would qualify for income support and a carer's premium might be added to this. Mrs Maycroft qualified for attendance allowance at the higher rate as she needed 24-hour care.

The government has also set up the Independent Living Foundation, and those who receive attendance allowance can apply to its trustees for money to pay for help with caring. The fund is receiving applications at the rate of 1 800 a month and may eventually have to limit or 'cap' payments.

There will usually be a social worker available to community nursing teams who can support clients in making claims.

The joint visit

When Ann Wilson and Julia Robb arrived for their joint visit they found a significant deterioration in Mrs Maycroft's condition. She was obviously breathless even at rest and was sitting in bed, not in the armchair as Ann was accustomed to seeing her. Both nurses suspected that she had a chest infection. Mrs Maycroft had simply accepted this deterioration as part of her condition, but Ann explained that it would be a good idea to ask Dr Anderson to visit as she should not simply accept these symptoms. It seemed that Mrs Maycroft was reluctant to admit that her pain had increased, but as Julia Robb subtly changed the question to ask about 'discomfort' it became clear that Mrs Maycroft's current analgesia was not very effective.

A further outcome of this visit was that the lymphoedema in Mrs Maycroft's arm was increasing and contributing to her discomfort. Julia Robb would therefore supply a glove and sleeve to ease this and the provision of a Spenco mattress for the bed also seemed appropriate. The application for Attendance Allowance under the special rule was moving forward and Mrs Betts should begin to receive this shortly.

Julia Robb also took the opportunity to explain to Mrs Maycroft and her daughter about the flexible arrangement her team had with the hospice, where breaks could often be arranged at short notice. The hospice had a day centre so another option would be for Mrs Maycroft to have day care from 10am to 4pm two or three times a week.

As the nurses had suspected, Mrs Maycroft did have a chest infection. Furthermore, as the X-ray ordered by Dr Anderson (and carried out at the local outpatients department) confirmed, Mrs Maycroft had secondaries in her lung. Despite this news, the few weeks before Christmas were positive ones for the family. Mrs Maycroft's analgesia was changed to diamorphine 2.5mg every four hours. The chest infection responded well to antibiotics and neighbours and friends rallied round. Although Mrs Betts had done a lot of her present-buying by catalogue, when the health visitor rang to say that one of the mothers from the mother and toddler group that she used to attend would be willing to look after the children for a couple of afternoons, Mrs Betts gladly accepted the offer.

Christmas was hectic at times because of the children's excitement but, as Judy Betts explained to Ann, while watching Emma picking up the cards and taking them to her grandmother for opening, 'I know this is where Mum should be'.

Mrs Maycroft was now very comfortable with Ann and always took advantage of the time her dressing was being changed to discuss her worries. She had been wondering what effect her illness and death would have on Emma.

Palliative care nursing

Palliative care nurses often plan a programme of structured activities aimed at preparing children for the death of a loved one and they might take on several follow-up visits after the death. Overleaf we see how compiling a scrapbook was used to help Mrs Betts' children relate to the illness of their grandmother. Other activities for such scrapbooks might be drawing simple face shapes to express feelings such as sadness, anger or happiness, and relating these to their own feelings. Older children can draw body outlines and shade in the body parts of their relative which they believe hurt them.

The following schedule outlines four follow-up visits carried out by a nurse in a support team for the dying in London (from discussions with Bloomsbury and Islington Health Authority's support team nurses, Myfanwy Jones and Jill Highat). The two girls, aged 8 and 10, had just lost their mother from breast cancer. Notice the forward planning in

Mrs Maycroft and Mrs Betts were shown a scrapbook designed by hospice staff which aims to help children relate to illness and death while feeling safe. The children were then encouraged to make their own giant scrapbook entitled *My Book About Nana*, so that they could paste in photographs and drawings which simply told the story of Mrs Maycroft and their relationship with her, in the context of the family. They could also add in pictures of where they live, a happy event such as Christmas, or of their teacher, who was someone to share sad things with. They could list and draw all those who came to their home to look after their Nana, which helped them to make sense of what was happening in their world.

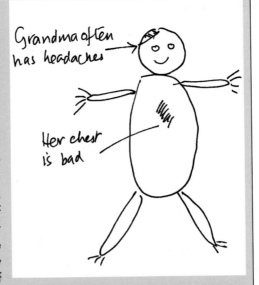

preparing the children for the termination of visits from the nurse, who had become a constant visitor to their home:

•**Visit 1** Look at the girls' thought diaries with them. School friend had said their mum would be dug up. Go through again why and how people die, and correct myths. Make card with them to take to the grave with Dad at the weekend. Leave them to complete their scrapbooks which they had looked at proudly several times during the visit.

Visit 2 Structured around the following activity: girls to draw a picture of how they see their family now and before their mother's death. Explore their coping mechanisms, now and into the future. Begin to face our separation.

Visit 3 Make a collage with pictures cut from magazines which represent happiness and sadness to the girls. Happiness included: my favourite pudding, Jesus, the cat, McDonalds and My Little Mermaid. Discussed the sadness of parting.

Final visit Having fun. The children chose from a list the activity they would most enjoy – an outing to the park and a visit to McDonalds. It was an opportunity to share all the work they had made and to say goodbye.•

It is likely that the nurse specialist or social worker would take on a bereavement follow-up programme like this one, but this is not always the case as resources often do not allow for such expertise to be available.

Postscript

It now seemed less realistic than a month ago for Mrs Maycroft to be left alone for any length of time and so with her agreement a plan was formulated that she would stay at the local hospice for a week in January to coincide with Emma's first week at school. The Christmas holiday went well. Some old friends from Mrs Maycroft's home town came to visit and Mr Betts was at home as the factory was closed until the New Year.

After Christmas the admission to the hospice went ahead as planned. Ann Wilson visited Mrs Maycroft at the hospice and she said that she was enjoying the 'bit of quiet time' that the break offered. However, towards the end of the week Mrs Maycroft developed another chest infection and the pain in her chest increased considerably, so symptom control was readjusted. However, despite this careful programme Lucy Maycroft died peacefully at the hospice on the Sunday that she was due to return home.

After Mrs Maycroft's death, Rebecca and Ann negotiated together who could most appropriately continue supportive visiting and bereavement work. It was important for there not to be duplication of effort which wastes the precious resource of community nurses. Equally, the family wanted only one nurse to co-ordinate continuing care.

Mrs Betts worried that the admission to the hospice had not been the best decision but, as Ann reminded her, Mrs Maycroft had been pleased to go there and was happy to be there.

After the bustle of the Christmas period Mrs Betts felt a strong sense of 'emptiness'. She said she was very glad that Emma had a nursery place as it gave them all a sense of purpose and some structure to their day. Emma made quite a friend of the nursery assistant and talked to her a lot about her grandmother.

Despite the sad aspects for Rebecca Johns and Ann Wilson of providing nursing support for the Betts family during Mrs Maycroft's terminal illness, there was also the challenge of helping them to achieve emotional growth during a period of crisis.

This case study has demonstrated some of the many facets of the work of a community nurse.

Community nursing practice is not for the 'quick-fix' merchant. The satisfaction and skills gained from nursing in a high-tech, speed-driven care setting, such as a high dependency unit, are a world away from the type of health care delivered by community nurses. Sometimes that care is continuous — as in Mrs Maycroft's case — while at other times the nurse may work with clients to resolve one aspect of their health care and then not actively participate in meeting further need until they identify that this is appropriate. There is also the challenge of working with people who are not sick but have other health needs, which involve lifestyle change.

Community nurse practitioners are skilled in identifying and responding to new health needs, such as 'give-up-smoking' sessions, or running a support group for women new to mothering. And every community — be it rural, market town or inner-city — has its own structure, culture and conflicts which are responded to by nurses working positively in each locality to reshape health in that environment.

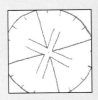

FOCUS
3 HOURS
Negotiate to follow up a patient who is being discharged from your practice setting. This should be done with the patient's consent and the knowledge of the ward manager and of the community agency receiving the referral.

Make your own observations of how successfully the discharge procedure went and then discuss the arrangements that were made with the patient herself and with the community staff involved. Discuss your findings with the other enrolled nurses in your study group, to ascertain their views of the discharge arrangements you described.

Add your findings to your community profile.

5.Politics, policies and trends in community nursing

In Section 1 of this module we discussed the link between demographic and social factors and health-care needs in the community, and in Sections 2-4 we looked at the role of the community nurse in meeting those needs. We have seen that these factors are creating a situation in which demand outstrips the resources available to pay for it in a state-provided health-care system, and it is this which forms the background to recent reforms in the health service.

We begin this final Section by looking at the political and economic factors which are changing the nature of the community health-care environment. You will, of course, be familiar with many of the issues raised in this Section, but we want to focus here on their particular impact for community nursing.

In the second half of the Section, we go on to explore ways in which community nursing is responding to these factors, and end by thinking about some of the trends which will shape community nursing in the future.

We have referred already in this module to some of the new measures which have been brought in to enable the state to meet the nation's health-care needs into the next century. We are going to consider here the impact of two pieces of legislation on community nursing:
• The NHS and Community Care Act 1990
• The Children Act 1989.

The NHS and Community Care Act 1990

The changes brought about by the NHS and Community Care Act represent the most radical change in health care in this country since the establishment of the NHS in 1948. The Act not only sets out to change the way the health service is organised and funded, it also sets out to change the way we think about health services at a very basic level.

The Act focuses on three main principles, which were set out in the White Papers *Working for Patients*[1] and *Caring for People*[2]:
• The establishment of a health-care market
• Increased consumer choice
• A switch in emphasis from institution-based care to community-based care.

The health-care market

To achieve a health-care market, new funding arrangements were agreed with district health authorities and those GPs who opted to become fund-holders. They became 'purchasers', and are given a budget with which to buy services. The purchasers draw up contracts which specify the amount and quality of health service they require to meet the needs of their local population, and the price they expect to pay. They then seek bids to fulfil their contract from 'providers'— local hospitals and community trusts or directly managed units — entering into negotiation with these bodies to obtain the best value for money.

The purchasers are responsible for assessing the health-care needs of their local population and ensuring those needs are met by arranging appropriate services, sometimes with a number of providers. Those providers who produce a plan which best matches the purchaser's requirements obtain the business. Providers who cannot match up may need to develop different plans in order to compete in the market or they may lose the business.

Producing a business plan is a valuable exercise for purchasers, as it makes every specialty or care group set out its priorities and development plans against the resources available, and allows them to take stock of how care is currently delivered. Providers will also be engaged in the business planning process, setting out specifications for the services they are able to provide.

Purchasers and providers work together closely. Their joint work is set out in the contract, which is the agreement which brings together the purchaser's requirements and the provider's commitments.

ACTIVITY 1
2-3 HOURS
Ask a community manager in your district for a copy of the current contract or service specification for the community nursing service. Read it through and imagine yourself to be a member of the purchasing team.

Pick out three strengths and three weaknesses in the quality of the nursing service. Look for evidence of:

• Evaluation of the effectiveness of the service
• Plans for new developments
• User views being sought
• Continuing education programmes.

Add the plan, and your evaluation of it, to your community profile.

Consumer choice
In implementing the NHS and Community Care Act 1990, the government also published *The Patient's Charter*[3] which sets out details of what users may expect in the delivery of health services. The Charter established the first nine national standards, including access to information, reduced waiting time and access to services, which will act as a benchmark of quality, and form a baseline for the development of local standards. Of particular importance for nurses is the standard which requires that a named qualified nurse, midwife or health visitor will assume responsibility for each patient's or client's care.

Whether we believe the Charter to be practical or impractical in our own area of work, it has heightened awareness both among health service consumers and health-care providers of the need to set acceptable standards of care, and find ways of ensuring that these standards are maintained.

If community nurses do not offer information about what their service offers and how people can access it, or do not ensure that home visits are booked at times to suit users rather than themselves, then consumers and purchasers may well look elsewhere.

The Patient's Charter is being developed at both national and local levels. The Department of Health has prepared a number of leaflets and publications on the subject; for example, *The Patient's Charter: the named nurse; The Patient's Charter: the named midwife; The Patient's Charter and family doctor services.* These are available free of charge from: *The Patient's Charter* Unit, Room 4N34B, Department of Health, Quarry House, Quarry Hill, Leeds LS2 7UE.

Community care
This third principle of the Act is dealt with in detail on page 69.

**ACTIVITY 2
1-2 HOURS**
Obtain a copy of your district health authority's local patient's charter. Read it and look for any references to community nursing services.

Discuss with the manager of your local community team the quality measures which are being used to assess standards in your local area .

The effects of the Act
The change to a purchaser-provider system and emphasis on consumer choice has led to a focus on the following principles in health-care management:
• Good quality care services
• Value for money
• Efficient use of resources.

We will now explore the impact of each of these on community nursing.

Quality and value for money: change in treatment methods
Change in traditional community nursing practice has often met with resistance, as some nurses feel that the pursuit of value for money inevitably reduces the quality of the service they provide. However, the need to demonstrate efficiency in the management of budgets has begun to bring about change in some areas. One authority[4] has already revolutionised the management of leg ulcers in the community.

Treating leg ulcers is one of the most difficult and frustrating aspects of the work of district nurses. It has been estimated that we spend £600 million a year nationally treating this condition[5].

In Riverside Health Authority a survey found that nearly half the district nurses expected leg ulcers to need treatment for between one and three years. But, with the introduction of four-layer, high compression bandaging, three-quarters of the patients' ulcers were healed after 12 weeks[4].

Riverside now has a system of leg ulcer care which has improved patient outcome, as well as district nursing skills, while achieving considerable savings.

ACTIVITY 3
2-3 HOURS
Find out what are the main dressings/products used for treating leg ulcers by district and practice nurses where you work. Why are these particular treatments chosen?

Reflect on whether you think district nurses in your area could benefit from reviewing their current practice for the treatment and management of leg ulcers.

Try to share the view you have developed with the district nurses you have been working with. If you can get hold of a copy of the journal describing the study[4], you could use the research evidence from that to support your case.

Value for money: skill mix
The major resource in community nursing is the time spent by nurses of various grades in managing, leading and providing care. In a climate of ever-increasing demand, managers need to be sure that they have the right balance of expertise (known as the skill mix) in the staff available to them, and that this expertise is used appropriately and efficiently.

Yet a report from the Audit Commission[6] found that few managers can explain why they have a particular number of G-grade nurses in the community, and a study by the NHS Management Executive's Value for Money Unit of three districts found G-grade nurses doing the same job as D and E grades, which it considered to be 'a gross waste of nursing resources, and failure to utilise the skills and potential of other nursing staff, both qualified and unqualified'[7].

This latter report recommended using G-grade nurses to conduct assessments, leaving the rest of the clinical work to other nurses and care assistants, and cutting the number of G and H grade posts by 50%[8]. It also recognised the need for more rigour in conducting caseload reviews, so that the service can be evaluated by asking questions about the number of clients seen, for how long, and to what effect by practitioners at different levels.

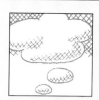

ACTIVITY 4
15 MINS
What do you think are the advantages and disadvantages of this approach to community care management for

• Clients?
• Community nurses?

Community nurses are expensively trained. They have the skills to head a team of support staff who can provide essential care to meet the needs of the growing numbers of older people, or people who have a disability, who require nursing services in the community.

Indeed, there is evidence that such community carers — a hybrid of a nursing auxiliary and a home help — have enabled frail elderly people to remain at home, and have reduced hospital admission of elderly 'at-risk' patients[6].

Community nurses have not resisted the growing use of non-professional support staff to carry out nursing and social care at home, and they recognise that it is important for them to be aware of how much their time is worth, and whether that time is being well spent. But there are two important issues which cause concern:

• If a community nurse decides, for example, that it is more cost-effective to send out for a take-away than to cook breakfast for a client at the weekend when the home help service is not available, she might miss a valuable opportunity to observe the client or to chat to him to discover information about other aspects of his care. A decision of this sort, on the actual value-for-money of time spent in carrying out community care tasks, requires a high degree of experience and skill, and cannot therefore be easily delegated to less-qualified practitioners.

• As we suggested in Section 2, the sort of collaborative planning by social services and health services required to replace the existing rigid and separate home help and nursing assistant services with a more unified range of health and social support has been slow to materialise, and until this type of provision is better developed, many community nurses feel that they are in the best position to ensure that appropriate care is received.

The criticisms in the two reports discussed above were in many ways redressed by a third report, *New World, New Opportunities*[9], which was published in 1993. This report stresses the importance of teamwork — both within the primary health-care team and with other agencies. It gives priority to the development of shared care initiatives, calling for joint strategies 'for the continuing care of elderly people needing sheltered care, and for joint services such as bathing and home help' (p 28, para 4.3).

The report also recommends that community nursing skill mix reviews should not be conducted in isolation from the overall task of using a team approach to provide for the identified needs of a defined population group. 'The main determining factor in skill mix in nursing should be the need for all professions to work together as a balanced complementary team to serve the population' (p 45, paras 14.6 and 14.7).

Resources: GPs and community nurses — practice in partnership

The health service reforms have also initiated changes in the nature of GP practice, which will have a direct effect on community nursing.

The first of these has given general practitioners a major role in purchasing health care. A fund-holding practice controls its own budget, and buys health-care that it cannot provide 'in house' on behalf of its patients. It is expected that non-fund-holders will be brought into the purchasing arena through FHSAs and DHAs.

The idea of 'locality purchasing' has been developed in *New World, New Opportunities*[9], which sets out a framework for bringing together community nurses, practice nurses, GPs and other health and social care providers. The aim is to be able to provide flexible, local primary health care for the population registered with each practice, and for practices to liaise both with other practices and with other bodies (such as community groups, local workplaces and housing trusts) to form healthy alliances which can provide exciting new forms of community health care.

The second major change in general practice has been the issuing of GP contracts which are aimed at improving patient choice and standards of primary care. Since 1990, the contract demands that GPs meet targets for screening for the early detection of unrecognised disease, and offer regular health checks to all practice clients over 75. Increasingly, all members of the practice team, and the community nurses who work with them, are involved in these activities.

There has been some controversy over the value of screening, and many practices are now developing comprehensive health promotion programmes which outline strategies and protocols for the whole team.

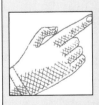

ACTIVITY 5
1-2 HOURS
You may wish to go back to the practice you studied in Section 2, and discuss the impact of the new GP contracts on the way the practice operates. In particular, you might like to concentrate on evidence of the formulation of shared goals and protocols by GPs and practice nurses.

These new approaches have meant many changes for community nurses, as well as GPs. There has been a large increase in the number of practice nurses since the introduction of the GP contract[6], providing a major new career opportunity for practitioners, many of whom are extending their role in line with the UKCC's *Scope of Professional Practice*[10].

Since April 1993, GP fund-holders have been able to negotiate contracts with other NHS providers to obtain a range of services, including community nursing. Practices are free to negotiate with a number of trusts and units to ensure a district nursing and health visiting service at an agreed price and quality. This development is enabling community nurses to become involved in the contracting process and to demonstrate the wide variety of services they can offer to GPs.

As with any major change, there are concerns that the new arrangements will not work as well as the old ones. There are particular worries that the increase in fund-holding and emphasis on the GP practice population may lead to some members of the community receiving a reduced service. It is for this reason that clear proposals for 'safety net services' and public health nursing have been set out in *New World, New Opportunities.*

ACTIVITY 6
1-2 HOURS
Arrange to discuss the implications of the GP contract with your local community nurses. What changes have they made, or are they making, to become involved in the contracting process?

We now turn to the third aspect of the 1990 NHS Act which has probably the furthest reaching implications for community nurses, the introduction of community care.

Community care

Caring for People[2], published in November 1989, proposed that local authorities would have the responsibility to purchase and manage packages of care for people who are elderly, mentally ill, have learning disabilities, or are disabled. The report argued that such vulnerable people and their carers deserved greater choice in their care, and, in particular, that alternatives to institutional care which allow people to be supported to stay at home should be developed.

We raised some important questions about community care in Section 1, and you might like to refer back to your diary to remind yourself of your thoughts on the subject at that stage of your work.

The important point about community care now is that it is a reality, and we need to consider the implications of this new approach to managing care for nurses in the community.

So how will community care work? Each local authority is to set priorities within available resources to agree who is eligible for social care services. The purpose of the new arrangements is to establish systems that ensure those in most need receive a swift and speedy response. Local authorities, working closely with health authorities, must ensure individuals know how to obtain an assessment of need.

A *care manager* (usually a social worker, but nurses are also being employed by local authorities to do this work) will carry out a comprehensive assessment, including an assessment of the person's financial means. The care manager will work out, with the customer, what services will best meet that person's need and what can be afforded.

Before April 1993, when the full effects of the Community Care Act came into force, the Department of Social Security would directly meet the cost of residential and nursing home care (whether in the public or independent sector) for those people whose low income would qualify them for social security payments at home. With the new arrangements, a sum of money is transferred to local authorities, who can then carry out assessments on an individual basis and use the allocated funds to arrange care. This may be in a residential or nursing home, or it may be a 'package' of care provided at home, or it may be a combination of home care and periodic respite care in a residential environment.

The important points are that the assessment is carried out at an early stage (for example, so that discharge from hospital may be planned well in advance), and that care arrangements are organised on an individual basis. Wherever possible, the consumer or client should be given a choice of services, and users and their carers should be involved in decision-making. National guidance on standards to be adhered to in this are laid out in the Department of Health/SSI document, *Guidance on Standards for Residential Homes for Elderly People*[11].

Care management can support people who wish to stay at home by designing imaginative packages of care to meet individual needs. Creative use of private domiciliary and day care services, for example, can offer cheaper ways of providing cleaning or shopping or personal freshen-up services to people. Use of Meals on Wheels is another example. Available since the last War, the service is widely used, often on a long-term basis, long after the original reason for using it has disappeared. If a person is only temporarily disabled, and cannot cook, then it may be more appropriate to provide some rehabilitative physiotherapy, and order a taxi to a local cafe or lunch club.

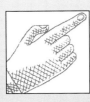

ACTIVITY 7
2-3 HOURS
Find out how community care is organised in your local area. If possible, make contact with someone who has been appointed as a care manager, and discuss how she sees her job developing as the community care changes are more widely implemented.

The care manager will not take over the role of a community nurse or general practitioner, who will contribute to people's assessment of care in the same way as before, but the principle of care being organised by just one person is important.

Carers have complained for years that a host of professionals filed into their homes, each conducting lengthy assessments of need and rarely involving the customer in the process. The result can be duplication of effort, and fragmented care.

The role of the community nurse in community care

Community nurses will contribute to joint care assessments, and in many instances they will take the lead assessor role where people require support from nursing services in order to remain at home. However, community nurses are aware that the distinction between health needs and social needs is often very blurred, and the question of who is the most appropriate person to assess and meet these needs may cause inequities.

For example, providing a bathing service for people who cannot manage this activity unaided is a responsibility which falls to nursing and social care providers. There is a clear distinction between a bath or shower which we all take independently or with assistance according to our level of dependency, and a bath which is provided by a qualified nurse with the direct intention of affecting a health problem in a positive manner. However, nurses are frequently called upon to provide a social bathing service, which is free at the point of provision, whereas a bath included in a care package arranged by social services may be charged for.

As we have suggested elsewhere in this module, the need for closer links between health and social service workers in the community is becoming more and more important as the community care reforms are implemented, and the speed and effectiveness with which such links are forged will be a significant element in their success.

Most authorities are optimistic about the benefits of the reforms, and joint training and collaborative working are presenting opportunities for workers in the health and social care fields to share their knowledge about people, and to understand one another's role.

ACTIVITY 8
3-4 HOURS
Ask for a copy of the new assessment documentation from your local social services department.

- Look at how the customers contribute to decisions about what they need
- Examine how unmet needs are recorded (for example, a carer may need regular breaks and, while it may not be possible to provide this, the fact that a need has been identified but not met should be recorded for future reference and planning purposes)
- If you have the opportunity, ask community nurses how they are being involved in the new assessment process.

Hospital discharge

Community care reforms will also have an impact on the quality of discharge planning, and will therefore affect the work of hospital-based nurses as well as community nurses.

For more than 20 years, hospital staff have arranged for elderly people to move directly on to independent sector homes. Now an assessment must be carried out first, and it is likely that more people with complex needs will return home with a care package arranged. A recent report[12] on elderly people's discharge from hospital found some people returning home to decaying food and unheated rooms. Often they were discharged within days of major surgery, irrespective of the age and health of their carers. The new arrangements for assessment, together with the development of individualised discharge protocols, should bring an end to such occurrences.

ACTIVITY 9
1 HOUR
Obtain a copy of your local general hospital's discharge protocol. Find the section on elderly patients, and consider:

• How elderly people and their carers are involved in the process
• How many days after discharge the ward team or liaison nurse contacts the patient to find out how the discharge has worked out
• How the community nursing services are involved in discharge planning and follow-up.

The Children Act 1989

The 1989 Children Act was introduced in response to problems involving liaison between health and social workers which came to light during a string of inquiries into child deaths at the hands of their parents or carers. This Act has had implications for many workers in the community, but in particular has affected the way health visitors work with families.

Before the Act was passed, health visitors often felt that their role in relation to children whose safety was causing concern was unclear. Health visitors have always covertly rationed their service by prioritising need and judging which of their clients need frequent supportive visits, and which can be supported by telephone calls and clinic visits. Sometimes they found themselves inventing excuses to visit families: 'I've just come to remind you that Kelly-Ann's check-up is due. How is she today?'

Under the Children Act 1989, health visitors now have a duty to assist the local authority in any investigation of a child at risk, and their role as key agents in promoting the welfare of children has been clearly acknowledged.

This has empowered health visitors to balance openly their first priority: to act on behalf of the child, against any accompanying intrusion of the child's parents, or potential damage to their relationship with the parents.

The interpretation of the Act has enabled health visitors to be more open with parents. Now, if health visitors have a concern about a child, they must raise this with the family and tell them that they intend to discuss the situation with social services.

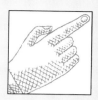

ACTIVITY 10
1 HOUR
The Children Act 1989 is an important piece of legislation which strengthens the rights of children and young people against abuse. It has relevance to all nurses, particularly those who work with young people.

If you are interested in this area, the Department of Health, in co-operation with the Royal College of Nursing, has produced a useful guide: *The Children Act 1989 — What every nurse, health visitor and midwife needs to know.* You can obtain a copy of it from: Health Publications Unit, No 2 Site, Manchester Rood, Heywood, Lancs OL10 2PZ.

This completes our review of the effects of recent legislation on community nursing. We want to end this module by looking to the future, and considering how these and other changes will affect the role of the community nurse into the next century.

Into the future

We started Section 5 by looking at social trends and health-care needs. As the NHS reforms are implemented, these trends will have some profound implications for the future of community nursing:

- The move towards more community-based care will continue, as hospitals increasingly become centres for the treatment of acute conditions in specialised, high-tech units

- People with progressive and degenerative disease will require increasing rehabilitative support from community nurses and the primary health care team

- The 'Hospital at Home' movement is expected to grow, as advances in health-care technology enable regular treatment for certain acute conditions, such as some end-stage HIV diseases, to be transferred to the home, if the patient so wishes

- The emphasis on prevention of ill-health and promotion of health, stimulated by the need to achieve national health targets, will involve all nurses in *The Health of the Nation* initiative.

All these factors will create a need for more widely-skilled and flexible community nursing staff, and the recognition of this fact has seen a flurry of investigative activity by various agencies into how these needs can best be met in the future.

The main findings of these investigations are discussed below, but you should plan to make time to read the reports themselves at some stage in your work on this module.

In 1986, the first major review of community nursing for over 30 years took place. *Neighbourhood Nursing: A focus for care*[13], commonly known as the Cumberlege Report, should be seen as another element in the wider NHS reforms of the 1980s, with similar objectives of overhauling management structures, improving the quality and efficiency of all health care services, including those in the community, and emphasising greater choice for people.

The major recommendations of the Cumberlege Report were the establishment of primary health care teams (as discussed in Section 2), and the formation of mixed teams of community nurses who would serve a defined population group.

The report argued that by bringing health visitors, district nurses and school nurses together, a more flexible, user-friendly, local team of nurses would be available to provide care in the community more efficiently and effectively.

The Cumberlege Report recognised that there are a variety of possible ways to organise community nursing services, and this view was reinforced in a more recent NHSME publication, *Nursing in the Community*[14], which set out five possible models for the organisation of community nursing in the context of primary health care. One of these models described the primary health care team approach to comprehensive care, reinforcing the policy set out in the government White Paper *Promoting Better Health*[15].

The Tomlinson Report in 1992[16] was particularly concerned with the development of health services for the people of London. It recommended that resources be diverted from the hospital sector to the community, to enable people to be treated more frequently by primary care services.

The development of London's community services has posed special challenges to the NHS and social services. High-density, multi-cultural, mobile population groups accustomed to living within easy reach of highly specialised hospitals have different expectations, and make different demands on those services than elsewhere in the United Kingdom. Plans for the development of London's health services were published early in 1993, in *Making London Better*[17] and a special group, the London Implementation Group, was set up to implement them.

London's special challenges are stimulating some exciting new developments in community nursing. Tomlinson recommended alternative methods of delivering primary care, citing the Lambeth Community Care Centre as an example of good practice.

In this small, community-based hospital, clinical responsibility rests with the GP on a 24-hour basis, with care carried out by a multidisciplinary team. The co-ordinating key worker is frequently a nurse. The Lambeth Centre, like other similar centres and community hospitals in the UK, can offer respite or palliative care, and treatment on a short-stay basis for people who prefer local care. It has also arranged for consultants to run 'outreach' clinics in the Centre, as a means of ensuring specialist treatment and care is locally available. Similar schemes are being tried in several other primary care locations nationwide.

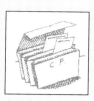

ACTIVITY 11
1-2 HOURS
Contact a community hospital in your area and find out if it has any arrangements similar to those described above for the Lambeth Centre.

Add your findings to your community profile.

Developing new approaches to primary health care and community nursing is the theme of *New World, New Opportunities*, the most recent government report on community nursing, which we have already mentioned in this Section. Launched in March 1993, the report reflects the many developments in the organisation and delivery of health-care services. It establishes a framework for the continued development of primary health care teamwork, and the accountability of primary health care and community nurses and their professional colleagues for the provision of services for the local population.

The report recognises the diversity of current developments, and refrains from making rigid recommendations. Instead, the task group which developed the report, chaired by Yvonne Moores, chief nursing officer, set out 12 cardinal principles that underpin primary health care nursing, and a large number of 'Keys to progress' to enable progress towards a multi-professional primary care service. *New World, New Opportunities* emphasises the chances that community nurses have to take a lead in developing new approaches to practice, 'enhanced by the freedom the new contract culture of the NHS has given providers'.

Many of the 'Keys to progress' are specific to nurses, and are captured in the mnemonic 'onstream': Opportunities for Nurses through Support, Teamwork, Research, Education, Audit and Management. The way in which community nurses use these 'keys' in their own specific area of practice will help to shape the pattern of primary health care in the future.

The reports we have been discussing in this final Section have raised other issues which are now being debated in community nursing:

Nurse practitioners
One change which is already under way is the increasing number of nurses who are developing the nurse practitioner role, and diagnosing and treating some common conditions which are more usually managed by a GP. Nurse practitioners in the UK are following in the footsteps of nurses in other countries who have developed this role. For example, in the United States, the management of chronic illness, health maintenance and promotion programmes are commonly led by nurse practitioners who have undertaken additional advanced preparation for practice.

In the United Kingdom, the South East Thames Regional Health Authority has established 20 pilot nurse practitioner projects[18]. The nurses taking part are studying the RCN's nurse practitioner course and, in accordance with legislation passed, will be able to prescribe a limited number of items, such as dressings, within carefully defined protocols, so that they can treat people independently. Such schemes, if they are considered successful and become more widespread, could allow real choice for members of the public, and enable the provision of primary health care for people who have difficulty accessing GP services, such as some travelling families, those who are homeless and those who are out at business all day.

There is some controversy about the use of the title 'nurse practitioner'. However, there is general agreement about the value of enhancing the role of all nurses, whether they practise in hospitals or in the community, and it is to this that we turn to end this module.

Community nurse training

As you will know, the UKCC has undertaken a major review of post-registration education and practice, including community nurse education. *The Post-Registration Education and Practice Project* report (PREP)[19], and the *Community Education and Practice (*CEP) report[20] will, following consultation, be formulated into final proposals.

The most significant of these in the short term are that all nurses and health visitors should maintain effective registration with the UKCC by engaging in a minimum of five days study every three years, and that a long career break should be followed by a return-to-practice course. Community nursing requires preparation beyond registration, and the latest UKCC proposals indicate that there should be particular areas of preparation for practice in relation to client need - for example, adults, children, learning disabilities, community health. These proposals differ from those outlined in the CEP report, and there is some concern that they will not meet the needs of all primary health care and community nurses such as practice nurses who treat and care for people of all ages, and with a variety of health needs.

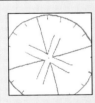

FOCUS
1-2 HOURS
Think about the enormous changes which are currently taking place in community nursing, and try a little crystal-ball gazing.

Imagine yourself as a nurse in the community in 10 years' time, and ask yourself the following questions:

- How will the changes we have been discussing in this Section influence the role of the community nurse and the environment in which she practises over that period?

- What differences might you envisage in Figures 1 and 2 on pages 26 and 27 of this module?

SECTION 5

References

1. Care in the community

1   Homecare. Going according to plan or going by default?[editorial] *At home: The Newsletter for Homecare Therapy Initiatives* 1992: September; 4, 1.
2   Roberts, P. Hip home. *Nursing Times* 1988: **188**: 44, 28-30.
3   Audit Commission. *Homeward Bound: A new course for community health*. London: HMSO, 1992.
4   Department of Heath. *On the State of the Public Health*. London: HMSO, 1991.
5   Bamford, O., Sparrow, S. A virtue in uniformity. *Nursing Times* 1990; **86**: 41, 46-48.
6   Laidman, P. *Health Education Research Report No. 12: Health Visiting and Preventing Accidents to Children*. London: Health Education Authority, 1987.
7   Luker, K., Orr, J. (eds). *Health Visiting*. Oxford: Blackwell, 1985.
8   Black, D. *Inequalities in Health*. London: Department of Health and Social Security, 1980.
9   Whitehead, M. *The Health Divide: Inequalities in Health in the 1980s*. London: Health Education Authority, 1987.
10 Watt, G.C.M., Ecob, R. Mortality in Glasgow and Edinburgh: a paradigm of inequality in health. *Journal of Epidemiology and Community Health* 1992: **46**: 498-505.
11 Rae, J.H. *Social Deprivations in Glasgow*. Glasgow: Glasgow District Council, 1975.
12 Jarman, B. Identification of underprivileged areas. *British Medical Journal* 1984; **286**: 705-709.
13 Jones, G.M. Elderly people and domestic care. *British Journal of Criminology* 1987: **27**: 2, 191-201.
14 Central Statistical Office. *Social Trends No. 22*. London: HMSO, 1992.
15 Brindle, D. Homes ruling shock for community care. *The Guardian* 1990: November 6.
16 Pitkeathley, J. Carers' concern. *Nursing Times* 1989: **85**: 31, 21.
17 McEwan, E. *Home Help and Care - Rights, Charging and Reality*. London: Age Concern, 1992.
18 Ewles, J., Simnet, 1. *PromotingHealth: A practical guide to health education*. Chichester: Wiley, 1985.

2. Organising care in the community

1   World Health Organisation. *Primary Health Care: Report of the International Conference on Primary Health Care, Alma-Ata, USSR*. Geneva: WHO, 1978.
2   Welsh Office. *Nursing in the Community: A team approach for Wales. Report of the Review of Community Nursing in Wales*. Cardiff: Welsh Office Information Division, 1987.
3   Department of Heath and Social Security. *Promoting Better Health. The government's programme for improving health care*. London: HMSO, 1987; Cmd 249.
4   Hocking, E. British Geriatrics Society. *Abuse of Elderly People. The Guardian* 1990: May 10.
5   Enfield & Haringey FHSA. *Guidelines on Pay Grades and Job Descriptions for Practice Nurses*. Prepared by Meradin Peachey, Nurse Adviser, January 1992.
6   Greenfield, S., Stilwell, B., Drury, M. Practice nurses: social and occupational characteristics. *Journal of the Royal College of General Practitioners* 1987; **37**: 341-345.
7   Department of Heath. *The Health of the Nation*. London: HMSO, 1992.
8   Barber, H.J., Kratz, A. *Towards Team Care*. Edinburgh: Churchill Livingstone, 1980.
9   Gilmore, M. *The Work of the Nursing Team in General Practice*. London: Council for the Education and Training of Health Visitors, 1974.
10 Department of Heath and Social Security. *The Primary Health Care Team: Report of*

a joint working group of the standing medical advisory committee and the standing nursing and midwifery committee. London: DHSS, 1981.

[11] Audit Commission. *Homeward Bound: A new course for community health.* London: HMSO, 1992.

[12] Hicks, D. *Primary Health Care Review.* London: HMSO, 1976.

[13] Bebbington, A., Charnley, H. Community care for the elderly - rhetoric and reality. *British Journal of Social Work* 1990; **20**: 410-432.

[14] Brent Area Health Authority. *A Child in Trust: The report of the panel of inquiry into the circumstances surrounding the death of Jasmine Beckford.* London: London Borough of Brent, 1985.

3. Setting priorities in community health care

[1] Audit Commission. *Homeward Bound: A new course for community health.* London: HMSO, 1992.

[2] Jarman, B. Identification of underprivileged areas. *British Medical Journal* 1984; **286**: 705-709.

[3] Dowlings, S. *Health for a Change.* Cambridge: Child Poverty Action Group in association with the National Extension College, 1983.

[4] Morton, S. Health and homelessness. *Health Visitor* 1990: **63**: 6, 191-193.

[5] Twinn, S. The heart of the matter. *Nursing Times* 1990: **86**: 32, *Community Outlook* (August), 11-14.

[6] Cross, A., Potrykus, C. Team spirit. *Health Visitor* 1990: **63**: 6, 188-189.

[7] Thorpe, L. *Shopping for Food.* Cardiff: Welsh Consumer Council, 1990.

[8] Laidman, P. *Health Education Authority Research Report No 12: Health Visiting and Preventing Accidents to Children.* London: Health Education Authority, 1987.

[9] Department of Health. *The Health of the Nation.* London: HMSO, 1992.

4. Delivering and planning home care

[1] Higginson, I., Wade, A., McCarthy, M. Palliative care: views of patients and their families. *British Medical Journal* 1990; **301**: 227-281.

[2] Copperman, H. Domiciliary hospice care: a survey of general practitioners. *Journal of the Royal College of General Practitioners* 1988; **38**: 411-481.

[3] Barker, W. *Child Development Programme. Early Childhood Development Unit.* Bristol: Senate House, University of Bristol, 1984.

[4] Clark, J. Delivering the goods. *Nursing Times* 1985; **81**: 2, *Community Outlook* (January) 23-28.

[5] Ross, F. *Recent Advances in Nursing: Information-Sharing Between Patients, Nurses and Doctors: Evaluation of a drug guide for old people in primary health care.* London: Churchill Livingstone, 1988.

[6] Lawon, B. The quiet revolution. *Primary Health Care* 1993; **3**: 5, 25.

[7] Hicks, D. *Primary Health Care Review.* London: HMSO, 1976.

[8] Department of Health and Social Security. Steering Group on Health Services Information. *A Report on the Collection and Use of Information about Services for and in the Community in the National Health Service.* Chair: Edith Körner. London: DHSS, 1984.

[9] Smith, S. Immunisation Facts Pack. *Community Outlook* 1991; **1**: 1, 16-17.

[10] Department of Health, Scottish Home and Health Department & Department of Heath and Social Security (Northern Ireland). *Immunisation Against Infectious Disease.* London: HMSO, 1992.

[11] Hart, M., Hedley, R., Rann, I. *Caring for Carers: A Survey by the Sunday Times and Crossroads Care Highlighting the Urgent Need for Better Facilities and Support.* London: Association of Care Attendant Schemes, 1990.

5. Politics, policies and trends in community nursing

[1] Department of Health. *Working for Patients.* London: HMSO, 1989.

[2] Department of Health. *Caring for People.* London: HMSO, 1989.

[3] Department of Health. *The Patient's Charter.* London: HMSO, 1991.

[4] Moffatt, C.J., Franks, P.J., Oldroyd, M., et al. Community clinics for leg ulcers and impact on healing. *British Medical Journal* 1992; **305**: 6866, 1389-1392.

5   Thomas, S. Cost-effective management of leg ulcers. *Nursing Times* 1990; **86**:11, *Community Outlook* (March), 21-22.

6   Audit Commission. *Homeward Bound: A new course for community health.* London: HMSO, 1992.

7   National Health Service Management Executive Value for Money Unit. *The Nursing Skillmix in the District Nursing Service.* London: HMSO, 1992.

8   Cost-cutting schemes halve district jobs [news]. *Nursing Times* 1992; **88**: 46, 5.

9   National Health Service Management Executive. *New World, New Opportunities.* London: HMSO, 1993.

10 United Kingdom Central Council for Nursing, Midwifery and Health Visiting. *Scope of Professional Practice.* London: UKCC, 1992.

11 Department of Health/SSI. *Guidance on Standards for Residential Homes for Elderly People.* London: HMSO, 1990.

12 Neill, J. Williams, J. *Leaving Hospital. Elderly people and their discharge to community care.* Report to the Department of Health. London: HMSO, 1992.

13 Department of Health and Social Security. *Neighbourhood Nursing: A focus for care. Report of the Community Nursing Review* (Cumberlege Report.) London: HMSO, 1986.

14 National Health Service Management Executive. *Nursing in the Community.* London: HMSO, 1991.

15 Department of Health. *Promoting Better Health: The government's programme for improving primary health care.* London: HMSO, 1987.

16 Department of Health. *Report of the Inquiry into London's Health Service, Medical Education and Research.* (Tomlinson Report.) London: HMSO, 1992.

17 Department of Health. *Making London Better.* London: DoH, 1993.

18 South East Thames Regional Health Authority. *Nursing in South East Thames. Nurse Practitioner Projects* 1992-4. London: SETRHA, 1992.

19 United Kingdom Central Council for Nursing, Midwifery and Health Visiting. *The Report of the Post-Registration Education and Practice Project.* London: UKCC, 1990.

20 United Kingdom Central Council for Nursing, Midwifery and Health Visiting. *Report on Proposals for the Future of Community Education and Practice.* London: UKCC, 1991.